How to Win at Quitting Smoking

VJ Sleight

Tobacco Treatment Specialist

Published by Stop Smoking Stay Quit

La Quinta, California

2015

ISBN: 978-0-9908629-0-1

PNC: 2014922320

ATTN: QUANTITY DISCOUNTS ARE AVAILABLE TO YOUR COMPANY, HEALTHCARE OR NON-PROFIT ORGANIZATION

For more information, please contact the publisher at:
Stop Smoking, Stay Quit
PO Box 5487
La Quinta, CA 92248
760-333-1270

VJSleight@cs.com

Dedication

This book is dedicated to the memory of the 480,000 Americans who die each year from tobacco. My hope is that someday no one needs suffer from the disease, disability and destruction of tobacco.

Table of Contents

Congratulations Letter from Author 1

How to Use This Book 3

Step One: Build Motivation 7

Have Good Reasons to "Become Smoke-Free" 7

*Make two lists, Benefits of "Becoming Smoke-Free", Figure out
how much money you will save, Consequences of "Continuing
to Smoke", Carrots or sticks, "Reasons to Quit" card*

Learn Why You Smoke 17

*Reasons for Smoking: Stimulation, Boredom, Something to do
with your hands and sensory pleasure, For the enhancement
of pleasurable feelings and to relax, Reward, Social situations,
Reduce stress and negative emotions, Relieve pain, Nicotine
dependency/physical craving, Habit, Figure out your number
of lifetime puffs, Tobacco use record*

Discover Your Obstacles to Success 33

*Nicotine dependence, Nicotine blood levels, Take the nicotine
dependency test, Reasons why cessation medications don't work,
Decide how to handle nicotine withdrawals, Beliefs, Answer the
following: I smoke because of positive reinforcement, or to avoid
negative consequences, Fear, Loss of approval, Loss of control,
Loss of enjoyment, Uncover your underlying fears, Releasing
fear meditation*

Reframe Your Obstacles to Success 49

*Make two lists, "Benefits of Smoking", "Consequences of
Quitting", Reframe beliefs and fears, Commitment, Compare
and contrast lists*

Challenge for Step One 58

Step Two: Create Your Action Plan 59

Set a Quit Date 60

Set a Quit Date, Spontaneous quit, Figure time spent smoking

Make a Personalized Action Plan 63

Make a smoking corner, Smoke by the clock, Track your common triggers, Action Plan, Toolbox approach

Countdown to Quit Day 69

Decide on preparation strategies: Get ready physically, Mentally, Change behaviors and manage your environment, Find support, Social support, Professional support, Closet smokers, Saboteurs, Make a list of support people

Challenge for Step Two 83

Step Three: Your First Smoke-Free Week 85

What to Expect 85

Physical withdrawal, Develop strategies for coping, Recovery symptoms, Nicotine withdrawal and coping strategies card

How Fast Your Body Heals 92

After 20 minutes, 8 hours, 24 to 72 hours, 1 to 2 weeks, 1 month to 1 year, 5 years, 10 years, 15 years

Reminders for Your First Week 94

You always have a choice, Five steps to train your brain

Challenge for Step Three 97

Step Four: Prevent Relapse 99

Understand Relapse 100

Difference between a slip and a relapse, Short-term relapse, Long-term relapse, Your reason for a previous relapse

Long-Term Maintenance 105

Emotional triggers, Handle stress without smoking, How stress affects your body, mind, emotions and behavior, How to relieve stress, Become stress-hardy, Reframing your attitude, Develop tools to change your attitude, ABCD method to reframe your thoughts, Avoid weight gain

Develop an ICE Plan 123

*Identify early warning signs, Identify high risk situations,
Create your ICE Plan, If you are smoke-free, If you have
relapsed, What does not work, If you haven't quit*

Challenge for Step Four 130

Appendices:

A: Assess Your Nicotine Dependence 133

B: List of Resources 135

Free Services, Advocacy

C: Various Chemicals in Tobacco Smoke 137

D: Summary of Cessation Medications 141

*Nicotine Replacement Therapy, The Patch, Gum, Lozenge,
Nasal Spray, Inhaler, Combination Therapy, Bupropion,
Chantix, Second Line Medications: Nortriptyline, Clonidine,
Mecamylamine, Websites for cessation medications*

E: Unproven and/or Ineffective Products/Services...152

*Acupuncture, E-cigarettes, Hypnosis, Lobedia, NicBloc, Silver
Acetate, Silver Nitrate, Smokeless Tobacco or Snus, Welplex*

**F: Partial List of Interactions between
Medications and Smoking** 155

G: The Seven "D's" 158

*Drink Water, Deep Breathing, Do Something Else, Delay,
Discuss with a Friend, Distract your Thoughts, Don't Smoke*

H: List of Activities and Visual Aids 162

About the Author 165

Congratulations!

You are about to do one of the best things you can do for yourself and for the people around you: *Become smoke-free*. It may be one of the hardest things you ever do in your life as well as being one of your most satisfying accomplishments. Quitting is not a one-time event where you just put your cigarettes down and walk away. It is a step-by-step relearning process. At one time you had to learn how to smoke, now you need to relearn how to live smoke-free.

As a former smoker, I know how difficult it can be to quit and what a hold cigarettes can have on your life. If you're like most smokers, you started as a teenager and smoking became associated with many parts of your life, and now the cigarettes control you.

Have you ever woken up in the middle of the night to find an empty pack, looked in the ashtray for a long butt, then driven to an all-night convenience store when you could not find a cigarette? Or missed an event because you knew you would not be able to smoke? Or hid your smoking from family, friends or your doctor to avoid their disapproving looks and comments? If so, then you know what I'm talking about when I say that nicotine has hijacked your life.

To take back your freedom and be successful, you need three things: First, you need to make up your mind that you really want to quit. Nothing can substitute for your own desire to be smoke-free. It requires your choice and commitment.

Second, you need the correct tools to help you through the quitting process and stay quit forever.

Third, you need to step out of your comfort zone and be willing to do things you have not done before, sometimes this won't be easy. There is no magic wand; instead, you'll find all the necessary tools within a systematic approach to overcoming the obstacles blocking your success.

> *"Magic is believing in yourself.*
> *If you can do that, you can make anything happen."*
> Johan Wolfgang Van Goethe

Once you are unshackled from smoking, you will experience a freedom like you've never known. Freedom from a nicotine addiction that has been controlling your life. You will be happier, less stressed and you'll wonder why you didn't stop years ago.

You are on your way to a new smoke-free you. It will be a journey of wonder and discovery that will lead to a better life for you and the people around you.

My thoughts and prayers are with you throughout your journey.

VJ Sleight, MA, Tobacco Treatment Specialist

How to Use This Book

Have you ever talked to a former smoker? They will tell you, *"If I can quit, ANYBODY can quit."* They can describe in great detail their long trial and error process of what they did to finally quit and what didn't work (implying it won't work for you either). But they are at the end of a journey that you are just starting. What worked for them may not work for you.

This drawn-out trial and error process can feel like putting a puzzle together with some of the pieces missing. Nothing fits together and you can't see the whole picture. This book is designed to shortcut your way by showing what pieces are missing in your plan to quit smoking.

This book has the exact information you need to walk through the difficult process of changing your identity from being a long-time smoker to being a former smoker. By following the step-by-step approach in this book, you expose the missing piece(s) in your quitting puzzle. You will find what methods will work for you instead of a lengthy trial and error approach or what worked for someone else.

As the pieces start fitting together, you will gain the confidence needed, find the necessary tools and develop the persistence required to be successful. This change is not always easy or quick, but I assure you it doesn't have to be painful and you *will* be successful.

However, if you only read this book without doing the activities asked of you or without answering the questions, you will gain information, but that will not change your behavior. There is no passive solution to an active problem. Just as you cannot learn to play a piano by reading a book, lasting change only happens by doing, especially something as difficult as becoming smoke-free. It is only by answering the questions and doing the activities that you will gain the personal knowledge to change your behavior. Information is worthless without action, so make a commitment to do what is asked and turn it into your personal experience. If your plan is to rely on willpower alone, that is almost a guarantee for relapse. By following the steps in this book, I guarantee it will shorten your journey to becoming a former smoker instead of relapsing.

This book is designed to make your transition as easy as possible, but everything is built on the work done from the previous steps. No matter how many times you have quit before or if this is your first time, start right at the beginning with the first activity. Don't skip any steps.

Buy a notebook. Write down your answers to the questions asked and the results of the various exercises. You will build on this information throughout the process and it is handy to have all the information in one place. The time spent thinking about the questions and the act of writing down your answers will help cement your commitment, confidence and motivation.

Find a "coach". Someone who will keep you accountable to spend time working towards your goal of being smoke-free. This could be a quit-buddy, a sponsor from Nicotine-Anonymous, a professional counselor, such as a Tobacco Treatment Specialist or an online support group.

Any time you feel strong anxiety or stress about quitting, it means you are getting too far ahead of yourself. Take a step back. View quitting not as a one-time event but a step-by-step process. So take your time and go at your own speed. Don't try to move from A to Z overnight. If it was easy you would have quit already. You have been smoking for many years—it takes time to change that imprinted behavior. Being successful means learning how to live every part of your life as a non-smoker. Be gentle with yourself. This is not a race; believe in progress, not perfection.

Let this be the *last time you quit,* not just the *next time you try;* remember—there is no failure until you stop trying.

"All great achievements require time."
Maya Angelou

"It does not matter how slowly you go
as long as you do not stop."
Confucius

Step One: Build Motivation

- Have Good Reasons to "Become Smoke-Free"
- Learn Why You Smoke
- Discover Your Obstacles to Success
- Reframe Your Obstacles to Success
- Challenge for Step One

"The starting point of achievement is desire."
Napoleon Hill

Have Good Reasons to "Become Smoke-Free"

Nobody wants to quit smoking. Nobody wants to give up the enjoyment of their cigarettes. But everyone successful at "Becoming Smoke-Free" has *wanted to* change their behavior, instead of feeling they *have to* quit. There is a difference between quitting something you enjoy (smoking) and truly desiring something else (Becoming Smoke-Free).

Motivation is your reason to do anything. Without a compelling desire, you won't put your full effort into making such a difficult behavioral change happen.

It is normal to be ambivalent and to have your desire come and go. On the one hand you want to be smoke-free but you also want to keep smoking. That is why it is important to remind yourself what you are working towards, not what you are giving up.

Transforming a behavior as resilient as smoking requires self-reflection and honesty about your feelings on change; acknowledging where you are, what you are willing to do, not where you *should* be and what you *should* do.

The key to lasting success is to build a strong motivational foundation of your relevant and personal reasons to "Become Smoke-Free"; to want this change for yourself and not because of pressure from friends, family or your doctor, who try to nag, shame or blame you into quitting.

The strongest motivation is when your behavior is in conflict with your values; when the use of tobacco does not fit the image of who you really are and what is really important to you.

Common values and/or principles: family values such as being a good spouse or parent, being a successful leader or role model for others, friendship, independence, freedom, acceptance by others, your good health or appearance, money, self-esteem, self-respect, peace of mind, integrity, truth, the environment, remaining physically active and able to participate in joyful activities.

Which of these values (or others) are important to you? If you had to pick either this value(s) or a cigarette, which one wins? Such as *"I can be a good parent or I can smoke but I can't have both"*. Include your values in your reasons to "Become Smoke-Free".

Activity: Make two lists, "Benefits of Becoming Smoke-Free" and "Consequences of Continuing to Smoke".

First, list your "Benefits of Becoming Smoke-Free"; what do you value? What is really important to you about "Becoming Smoke-Free"? Next, list your "Consequences of Continuing to Smoke". Keep adding new items to your lists as you uncover new benefits and consequences.

Benefits of Becoming Smoke-free	Consequences of Continuing to Smoke
1. Better Health	1. Health gets worse
2. Save Money	2. Spend more money
3. Good role model for kids	3. Bad role model
4. Spouse won't nag	4. Continued nagging
5. Dangers of secondhand smoke	5. Continued risk for loved ones
6. Smell better	6. Continue to stink
7. More energy	7. Fatigue
8. More time	8. Less time
9. Social Acceptance	9. Remain a pariah
10. No more burn holes	10. More burn holes
11. Keep my job	11. Might have to change jobs

Benefits of "Becoming Smoke-Free". Your "Benefits of Becoming Smoke-Free" need to inspire you, so always state your reasons as something positive:

"I will be in control of my life instead of the cigarette."

"I will live longer, be healthier and feel more physically fit."

"I will breathe better, cough less and walk without gasping for breath."

"I will participate more because I won't be outside smoking."

"I will be a better role model for my children and my family will be safe from secondhand smoke."

"I will smell better. Food will taste better."

"My clothes and furniture will be free of burn-holes."

"I can go on long trips and go to places where smoking is not allowed without trying to figure out where I can smoke."

"I will sleep better."

"I will improve my self-esteem and feel better about myself."

"If I can quit, I can do anything!"

Ask your doctor how "Being Smoke-Free" will benefit your physical health and ability to continue having an active lifestyle:

"My blood pressure and cholesterol will be lower."

"My breathing and my ability to walk or climb a flight of stairs will get better."

"My complexion will improve from increased blood flow."

"My medications will work more efficiently and I will be at a lower risk for side effects."

"My operation will have a better outcome, my body will heal faster and my recovery will be shorter."

"I want a complication-free pregnancy and a healthy baby."

"I will have a whiter smile, less cavities and healthier gums."

Activity: Figure out how much money you will save by not smoking.

"I will save a lot of money and spend less time having to drive to the store when I run out of cigarettes."

"My insurance premiums will be lower."

How much do you spend each day for cigarettes? If you and your spouse or partner both smoke, figure the amount for both of you.

Next, ask yourself: *"What other expenses do I have if I continue to smoke?"* (For example: lighters, ashtrays, burn-holes in clothes, breath mints/sprays and increased insurance premiums). *"If I don't quit now, how many more years will I smoke?"* Would it be reasonable to imagine that if you don't stop now, you might continue smoking for another five years?

Calculate how much you will save in one year and over five years if you quit now (or how much you will burn up if you continue to smoke).

Cost/day	1 year	5 years	Cost/day	1 year	5 years
$3.00	$1,095	$5,475	$10.00	$3,650	$18,250
$3.50	$1,277	$6,387	$11.00	$4,015	$20,075
$4.00	$1,460	$7,300	$12.00	$4,380	$21,900
$4.50	$1,642	$8,212	$13.00	$4,745	$23,725
$5.00	$1,825	$9,125	$14.00	$5,110	$25,550
$5.50	$2,007	$10,037	$15.00	$5,475	$27,375
$6.00	$2,190	$10,950	$16.00	$5,840	$29,200
$6.50	$2,372	$11,862	$17.00	$6,205	$31,025
$7.00	$2,555	$12,775	$18.00	$5,670	$32,850
$7.50	$2,737	$13,687	$19.00	$6,935	$34,675
$8.00	$2,920	$14,600	$20.00	$7,300	$36,500
$8.50	$3,102	$15,512	$30.00	$10,950	$54,750
$9.00	$3,285	$16,425	$40.00	$14,600	$73,000
$9.50	$3,467	$17,337	$50.00	$18,250	$91,250

Do you think cigarettes will get any cheaper? How much has the price increased since you started to smoke? How more will they cost in the future? When will your state increase the tobacco tax and by how much?

Consequences of Continuing to Smoke. The items on your second list are negative events, consequences you fear if you don't stop smoking. Perhaps they are your worst nightmare since smoking affects every system in your body:

- Cardiovascular system: diseases of the heart and blood vessels, stroke, aneurysm.

- Respiratory system: emphysema, chronic bronchitis, asthma problems.

- Reproductive system: difficulty achieving an erection, trouble getting pregnant, complications in pregnancy, premature births, low birth weight, sudden infant death syndrome (SIDS).

- Cancer: lip, mouth, throat, esophagus, voice box, lung, stomach, pancreas, liver, colon, kidney, bladder, uterus, cervix, breast and some types of leukemia.

- Other physical problems: wounds not healing, low bone density, stomach ulcers, eye diseases, diabetes, increased duration and severity of colds and the flu.

- Esthetics: wrinkles, pasty complexion, cavities, tooth loss, gum disease, bad breath, yellow teeth and fingers.

Ask your doctor what your personal health risks are if you continue to smoke. Your risk of harmful side effects of some medications may increase; such as smoking while using birth control pills increases your risk of a stroke or chemotherapy may not be as effective. These could be your consequences:

"I don't want to gasp for breath as I climb stairs."

"I don't want to have to cart around an oxygen tank."

"I don't want heart disease, cancer or a stroke. I don't want chronic obstructive pulmonary disease (COPD – emphysema and/or chronic bronchitis). I don't want diabetes."

"I don't want cataracts or macular degeneration."

"I don't want to have bronchitis every winter or be sicker from the flu or a cold since smoking makes it worse."

"My medications won't be as effective."

Ask your dentist or hygienist if they can tell a smoker by their teeth and gums. Consequences could be:

"I don't want yellow teeth, more cavities, gum disease or smoker's breath."

If you have small children, talk to their pediatrician about the effect secondhand smoke has on your family:

- Children and infants of smokers have an increased risk of developing asthma, lung and ear infections.
- Babies born to smokers are more likely to have learning problems, be more cranky and restless and get sick more often.
- Nonsmokers have an increased risk of heart disease and breathing problems, and will die younger than people who are not exposed to secondhand smoke.

"I don't want to harm my family and friends from the effects of secondhand smoke."

Secondhand smoke (environmental tobacco smoke) is the combination of the greyish white smoke you exhale and the blueish side-stream smoke coming off the tip of your cigarette when you hold it. Side-stream smoke is more harmful as it is formed at a lower temperature, producing more cancer causing chemicals than the smoke formed from when you inhale and pull smoke through the cigarette, which burns at a higher temperature causing the tip to flare up. Inhaled smoke is filtered by your body before you exhale but side-stream smoke is not, and both you and anyone within 20 feet inhale it.

Talk to your vet about the effects of secondhand smoke on your dog or cat. Pets of smokers are more likely to develop certain types of cancers. Dogs get cancer in their noses and cats get oral cancer from licking their fur which is covered in smoke residue.

"I don't want to be responsible for my pets getting sick."

There are many other unwanted "Consequences of Continuing to Smoke":

"I don't want my family to watch me die from a horrible disease or have to care for me if I should become disabled."

"I don't want to be the only one in my social group who smokes and have the social stigma of being a smoker."

"I don't want the cigarette to continue to control me or have to worry about where I will be able to smoke."

"I don't want any more burn-holes in my clothes, furniture or car, or catch my house on fire."

Carelessly discarded butts are the leading cause of fatal fires with property losses totaling hundreds of millions each year.

"I don't want to contribute to environmental trash or damage."

Cigarette butts are made of plastic fibers which can take 12 to 15 years to break down. Butts are a major component of trash in the US (135 million pounds annually), and account for up to half of the trash on the side of the road.

One in eight trees cut down worldwide go into the production of tobacco products. This is a leading cause of deforestation in the developing world.

There are 25 million pesticide poisonings per year due to tobacco production. About one quarter of tobacco workers have suffered green tobacco sickness at least once.

Carrots or Sticks. Two things motivate: working towards what is wanted are *carrots*, and moving away from or avoiding things not wanted are *sticks*. Carrots are pleasing, desirable and are more motivating because they evoke positive emotions. Sticks are unwanted, evoking a negative reaction which you want to ignore or deny.

Every statement on your list can be reframed either as a carrot or stick to maximize the motivating effect. Every negative outcome you want to avoid by continuing to smoke can be reframed as a positive reason to "Become Smoke-Free". Every positive reason to "Become Smoke-Free can be reframed as a negative outcome to avoid if you continue to smoke. See page 115 for more on reframing.

Choose whichever statement is more powerful, encouraging and motivating to you. For example: *"I want to be healthy."* Or, *"I don't want to get cancer or heart disease".*

"I want to save money to buy other things." Or, *"I don't want to waste more money on cigarettes."*

"I will smell better." Or, *"I will continue to stink."*

"I will be in control." Or, *"My cigarettes will continue to control me."*

"My relationship with my spouse will improve." Or, *"My spouse will continue to nag me."*

Activity: Make a Reasons to Quit Card.

Cut card stock paper into the size of a business card. On one side of the card, list your four most important carrots or motivating "Benefits to Being Smoke-Free". On the back side list your worst nightmares, the consequences you most want to avoid if you don't quit.

Reasons to Quit Card

Front Side	Back Side

Carrots: My Benefits of being Smoke-Free	Sticks: My Consequences of Smoking
1.	1.
2.	2.
3.	3.
4.	4.

Because you will work harder for the things you want, place your Reasons to Quit Card, with the carrot side facing out, between your cigarette pack and the outside cellophane.

Always read your carrots on your Card through the clear wrap, before you light up. This is a constant reminder of what is more important to you than a cigarette and what you are working towards. It also makes smoking a conscious decision instead of an automatic habit.

It is easy to minimize and rationalize away unwanted negative consequences, but your motivation can change. If your carrots don't seem motivating, take your Card out and read the back side which has the consequences you want to avoid, i.e. your worst nightmare.

Don't forget to take your Reasons to Quit Card out of your pack when you throw it away.

Learn Why You Smoke

Each cigarette you smoke can be for a different reason and every smoker has different habits, connections and associations with their cigarettes. This is why some methods work for some smokers and not for everyone. The reason you smoke a cigarette can vary and the tool used to avoid it needs to match the reason for smoking it.

Activity: Reasons for Smoking.

Read each of the following statements and decide which apply to you. Start thinking about which alternative suggestions you might try and write it down in your notebook. You will use these ideas when creating your Action Plan (see page 66).

Smoking for Stimulation. Nicotine is a stimulant. Smoking increases your heart rate and blood pressure.

Stimulation cigarettes:

"I smoke cigarettes in order to keep myself from slowing down, such as in the late afternoon."

"Smoking gives me an increased sense of energy."

"I smoke to get myself moving, or to perk myself up."

"I need a couple of cigarettes just to wake up in the morning."

"I smoke when I am tired to give myself a 'lift'."

"Smoking helps me to concentrate when I am reading, studying or working on the computer."

Alternatives: Find a different way of getting energized:

- Go for a brisk walk or other exercise.
- Take a cold shower or splash cold water on your face.
- Start a new stimulating hobby.
- Have a cup of coffee, tea, or energy drink.

Smoking Out of Boredom. Smoking fills up time. The average smoker spends more than one and a half hours a day smoking, which is over 22 days in a year.

Boredom cigarettes:

"Smoking gives me something to do to kill time and breaks the boredom."

"I smoke a lot when I am alone."

"I smoke when I have dead time on my hands."

"I smoke when I need a break or need some down time."

"I smoke when I'm lonely."

Alternatives: Plan ahead for when you have extra time on your hands. Examples could be:

- Take a magazine, book or e-reader with you wherever you go.
- Google yourself or play a computer game on your phone or tablet. Try a new one which challenges you and makes you think. When you are concentrating on something else you are not thinking about smoking.

- Think about all the things you can buy with the money you will save.

- Find a new hobby, take a class at the local community college. Start a second job or a home-based business.

- Always have your notebook with you and work on your Action Plan (see page 66).

Smoking for Something to Do With Your Hands and for Sensory Pleasure. Cigarettes have been designed to provide the most pleasure to all your senses. They just feel right in your hand. Holding one is like having a security blanket; it does not feel right when you are not holding a cigarette. Inhaling the smoke can be enjoyable. Menthol cigarettes can enhance the taste of coffee or alcohol.

Sensory cigarettes:

"I feel awkward when I'm not smoking because I don't know what to do with my hands."

"Cigarettes taste good. I like the cool taste of menthol."

"Handling a cigarette is part of the enjoyment of smoking; from packing the tobacco to lighting up and holding it in my hand."

"I like blowing smoke rings and watching the smoke as I exhale."

"I enjoy the feeling of the cigarette and the smoke on my lips and tongue."

"Coffee (or other beverage) doesn't taste the same if I'm not smoking."

"I love the smell of a cigarette when I first light up or have not had one in a while."

Alternatives: Find something to keep your hands and/or mouth busy without smoking. Don't use food as an oral substitute for a cigarette if you are concerned about gaining weight.

- Keep a pen and scratch pad handy. Doodle or sketch.

- Play with a coin, a piece of jewelry, silly putty, a pen or pencil. Get a stress ball to squeeze.

- Use a straw, coffee stirrer, toothpick, cinnamon stick, licorice root, or pretzel stick to replace holding a cigarette. Suck on sugarless candy.

- Play a musical instrument such as a harmonica.

- Switch to flavored coffee or add a sweetener.

Smoking for the Enhancement of Pleasurable Feelings and to Relax. The feeling of relaxation and enjoyment are caused by the flood of dopamine in the pleasure pathway of your brain. Dopamine is a natural chemical neurotransmitter and is responsible for *"I feel good"* sensation.

Relaxation cigarettes:

"Smoking is pleasant and relaxing."

"I enjoy smoking. It's fun."

"I light up a cigarette when I am most relaxed and comfortable."

"Smoking helps me relax quickly when I feel tense."

Alternatives: Learn other ways to relax without self-medicating with nicotine. Examples:

- Spend more time doing activities you enjoy where smoking isn't allowed.

- Take 10 slow, deep breaths for a calming effect. Learn to meditate. See pages 71 and 111 for other breathing and relaxation exercises such as progressive muscle relaxation.

- Understand the enjoyment you feel is just a reaction to the drug nicotine. Your level of enjoyment can indicate your level of addiction. Read about how nicotine affects your brain (see page 34).

Smoking as a Reward. After completing a task, smoking can feel like a reward.

Reward cigarettes:

"I smoke when I need a break."

"I smoke after completing a project or a household chore."

"I smoke as a reward when I want to feel good."

Alternatives: How much money did you calculate that you spend on cigarettes on page 10? Use that money to find new ways to reward yourself. Don't feel deprived when you quit—plan a reward by doing something nice for yourself for "Becoming Smoke-Free". Avoid using food as a reward. Better rewards:

- Buy a new magazine subscription, i-Tune, DVD, e-book or app.

- Get tickets for a concert, sports or cultural event.

- Take a golf lesson, exercise or yoga class.

- Have a massage, manicure or pedicure.

- Pay monthly dues at a health club.

- Go out to dinner at a special restaurant.

- Buy a new article of clothing.

- Invest in a hobby or gardening supplies. Buy flowers and enjoy their scent.

- Arrange a few hours of baby-sitting (free time for you).

New rewards don't need to be expensive and don't have to cost money:

- Sleep late on the weekend.

- Spend extra time on a hobby or activity you enjoy.

- Give yourself a pat on the back. Quitting is hard and you deserve credit for your efforts.

Smoking in Social Situations. Smokers often feel it enhances their pleasure in social situations and feel deprived of enjoyment when they quit.

Social cigarettes:

"I smoke at parties and other social events and when I'm celebrating or drinking alcohol."

"I smoke when I'm with other smokers. Most of my friends smoke; it's something we do together."

"I smoke at break time when I am talking to co-workers who also smoke."

Alternatives: Separate your smoking behavior from your feelings and realize you can still have a good time without smoking. You don't need to smoke just because others are.

- Avoid smoking areas and being around other smokers until they are no longer a temptation to smoke.

- If you can't avoid social situations where you might be tempted to smoke, take along your quit buddy (see page 82) or a non-smoking support person.

- Avoid alcohol at social events until it doesn't trigger a craving.

- Talk to your family and friends who smoke before you quit and ask for their help (see page 77).

- Practice saying *"no"* for times when you are offered a cigarette.

- Make new non-smoking friends. Seek out non-smoking acquaintances who will support you.

- Do something else, like go for a walk, on your break instead of going to the smoking area.

- Join a nicotine anonymous group, an on-line support group such as BecomeAnEx.org or a local anti-tobacco coalition.

Smoking to Reduce Stress and Negative Emotions. Most smokers use tobacco ease their stress but actually smoking increases the stress in your life. Former smokers report less stress after quitting. See Step Four, Handle Stress without Smoking on page 108 for more ideas. It may be easy to quit when things are going well, but without new coping skills, you may be tempted to have "just one" in times of extreme stress.

Stress cigarettes:

"I light up when I am trying to solve a problem."

"I smoke when I feel blue, uncomfortable, or I'm upset about something. Nothing helps me feel better than smoking a cigarette when I'm upset."

"I smoke when I want to take my mind off of my cares and worries."

"I light up when I am angry, irritable, frustrated or get in an argument with friends, family or coworkers. Smoking calms me down."

"When I am faced with difficulties of any kind, smoking seems to make it easier to face my troubles."

Alternatives: Stress is a major cause of relapse because most smokers have been using cigarettes as their main source of coping since they started to smoke as a teen. Those who have never smoked, have never depended on cigarettes as a crutch and have developed other ways of coping which you now need to learn.

These new coping methods to manage stress may require more effort than you are used to, which is to just light up:

- Be aware of stressful situations and visualize yourself handling the situation without smoking.

- Plan ahead. Think how you will handle stressful situations during the day without smoking. Ask former smokers what they do now for stress instead of smoking.

- Tell yourself that smoking isn't going to make the situation any better and may actually make it worse since you might relapse.

- Attend a class on mindful meditation, assertiveness training or stress management. Learn relaxation exercises such as progressive muscle relaxation (see page 111).

- Take a time out. Call a friend and talk it out.

- When feeling irritation and anger, don't hold it in but let it out. Hit a pillow, go for a walk or go to the gym and exercise it out.

- Discuss the use of medications with your doctor. Some stress you experience is really caused by nicotine withdrawal. Bupropion is also an anti-depressant and may help with negative emotions.

Smoking to Relieve Pain. Smoking releases dopamine and can be a type of self-medication. In some situations, smoking makes your physical pain worse. It can mask a serious physical problem by reliving a pain that should be alerting you that something is wrong.

Pain relief cigarettes:

"I take less pain medication when I smoke."

"My pain is worse when I'm not able to smoke."

"Whenever I quit smoking, I get pains in my . . ."

Alternatives: Other options are:

- Work with your doctor to adjust your pain medications. Discuss the use of nicotine replacement products for pain reduction. If you develop new pain after quitting, see your doctor.

- With the advice of your doctor, try complementary pain relief such as: acupuncture, self-hypnosis, biofeedback or meditation. Apply ice or heat. Take a warm bath, sit in a Jacuzzi or hot tub. Have a massage or try stretching.

Smoking out of Nicotine Dependency/Physical Craving. Nicotine is an extremely addictive drug causing intense cravings and other physical withdrawal symptoms (see page 86). See page 34 to read about how nicotine has affected your brain. To assess your nicotine dependence see page 133.

Dependency cigarettes:

"I smoke a pack a day or about one an hour."

"I smoke within 30 minutes of getting up in the morning."

"I am very much aware of the fact when I am not smoking a cigarette."

"I get a real gnawing hunger for a cigarette when I haven't smoked in a while."

"If I run out of cigarettes, I find it almost unbearable until I can get them."

"I continue to smoke even though I find the taste unpleasant."

"I've never been able to stop for more than a day or two."

Alternatives: Ways to reduce cravings:

- Drink plenty of water or citrus juice to flush your system.

- Do deep breathing exercises, (see pages 71 and 111).

- The craving will pass whether or not you smoke. Find a way to wait it out. Delay by changing your activity, count to 300 or set the clock and wait five minutes then get your mind on something else.

- Exercise. Take a short walk.

- Make sure no cigarettes are around.

- Avoid friends who smoke until they are no longer a temptation.

- Call a supportive friend.

- Take a shower.

Smoking as a Habit. Habits are a "conditioned response" or pattern, in the form of a trigger – then a response. The most famous example of this is from the scientist, Pavlov, who conditioned dogs to salivate when they heard a bell ring. The trigger was a bell, and their response was to salivate. Nicotine trains the automatic nervous system in your brain to react in the same involuntary and unconscious manner. It is the reward center of your brain where an automatic behavior, like smoking, becomes connected to the pleasurable effects from the release of dopamine.

When a trigger is present you reach for a cigarette with no thought or feeling attached. With enough repetition almost anything can become a trigger for a craving. Trigger – activities, places, situations, people, feelings or times; your response is always the same – you light up. Just as Pavlov's dogs expected to get food when they heard a bell ring, your brain expects to get nicotine whenever you are around one of your triggers.

The key to success is to become aware of each cigarette you smoke instead of acting out of an unconscious habit.

Habit cigarettes:

"I smoke when I'm watching TV, reading, or when I'm on the computer playing games, checking e-mail or on Facebook."

"I always smoke in certain situations such as answering the phone, driving, with coffee/tea/soda/alcoholic drink or after a meal."

"I smoke automatically without even being aware of it. I have found a cigarette in my mouth and didn't remember putting it there or I have lit up and then found one already burning in the ashtray."

"There are specific times during the day when I regularly smoke, such as with my morning coffee or driving."

"Right after lighting a cigarette, I put it out because I realize I don't really want it."

Alternatives:

- Replace old habits with new ones. Instead of having a cigarette, go for a walk.

- Ask yourself, *"Do I really want this cigarette or I am reaching for it out of habit?"*

- Make smoking a conscious choice. Start a Tobacco Use Record described on page 32.

- After meals: Go for a walk, brush your teeth, have a mint, wash the dishes by hand. Delay smoking after a meal by five minutes. Increase the length of the time-delay by five minutes each day.

- Driving in the car: Do something that mimics the hand-to-mouth motion of smoking. Eat unsalted, unshelled sunflower seeds or raisins, one at a time. Have a water bottle that you sip frequently. Use a cinnamon stick to hold in your hand and chew on.

- Answering the telephone: Only talk on the phone in a non-smoking room, such as the bedroom. Grab a pen and pad of paper to doodle while talking. Don't take your phone outside with you when you smoke. Make your phone calls short or don't answer it.

- Drinking coffee/tea/soda: Sit in a different chair when having your morning coffee. Change brands or flavors. Switch from coffee to tea. Switch to water or iced tea instead of a soda.

You know your common every day habits. What are some that are not ordinary? Think about different people, objects, places, times, emotions, events or situations where you *always* smoke that may only happen once in a while. What ideas do you have to counter those circumstances?

Activity: Figure out how many cigarette puffs you have smoked over your lifetime.

Habits are created by repetition. Each puff is a smoke signal to your brain to associate what you are doing or how you are feeling with smoking.

How many cigarettes per day do you smoke? In one year? For example: 20 cigarettes per day X 365 days = 7,300 cigarettes per year.

(Number of cigarettes per day X 365 days = the amount smoked for one year. See the upper left part of the chart).

Next calculate how many lifetime cigarettes you have smoked. Take your annual amount times the number of years you have smoked.

For example: 7,300 cigarettes smoked per year X 30 years = 219,000 lifetime cigarettes smoked.

(Annual amount X the number of years smoked. See upper right part of the chart).

Number of Cigarettes/Puffs Smoked per Day Over Time

Number of Cigarettes per day	Number of Cigarettes smoked per year	Over 10 years	Over 20 years	Over 30 years	Over 40 years	Over 50 years
10	3,650	36,500	73,000	109,500	146,000	182,500
20	7,300	73,000	146,000	219,000	292,000	365,000
30	10,950	109,500	219,000	328,500	438,000	547,500
40	14,600	146,000	292,000	438,000	584,000	730,000

Puffs per day	Puffs per year	Over 10 years	Over 20 years	Over 30 years	Over 40 years	Over 50 years
10 cigarettes = 100 puffs	36,500	365,000	730,000	1,095,000	1,460,000	1,825,000
20 cigarettes = 200 puffs	73,000	730,000	1,460,000	2,190,000	2,920,000	3,650,000
30 cigarettes = 300 puffs	109,500	1,095,000	2,190,000	3,285,000	4,380,000	5,475,000
40 cigarettes = 400 puffs	146,000	1,460,000	2,920,000	4,380,000	5,480,000	7,300,000

The average puffs per cigarette is about 10 puffs or 10 hits of nicotine. Now take your number of lifetime cigarettes smoked X 10 puffs.

For example: 219,000 lifetime cigarettes X 10 puffs = 2,190,000 lifetime puffs! (See lower portion of chart for puffs smoked: 20 cigarettes = 200 puffs per day over 30 years = 2,190,000 puffs).

So if you have smoked a pack a day for 30 years—that is over two million puffs! Can you think of anything else you do that often? It is this repetitive hand-to-mouth puffing and inhalation of nicotine which trains your brain to create automatic behaviors (habits) that are linked to all your other activities (triggers).

It may feel like your "habit" cigarettes are the hardest to break and you find it almost impossible to not smoke with some activities because these patterns feel so comfortable; actually they are the easiest because you get to practice every day.

It takes about three to four weeks, or about 30 consecutive actions to "break" a habit; or as Pavlov would say, *"the conditioning is extinguished"*. For example, if you smoke when drinking coffee, you will need to drink coffee without smoking about 30 times over three to four weeks before you will feel comfortable drinking coffee without a cigarette. Think of how many times you have smoked while having a cup of coffee over the years and realize you now need to repeat a new and different behavior many times to break that association. Have you (or someone you know) ever purchased a new car and not smoked in it? Before long you don't miss smoking in your car at all. In Step Two, you will learn how to break your habit cigarettes before you quit (see page 63).

Activity: Start a Tobacco Use Record.

To get to where you are going, you need to know where you are starting. If your destination is New York City, the route would be different whether you started in Seattle or Miami.

A Tobacco Use Record is a useful exercise to learn where you are starting. The more you know about your personal connections to smoking the easier it is to map out a Plan to where you want to go.

Before every cigarette, write down the time, place, how you are feeling or your reason for smoking, then rate the intensity of the craving from 1 to 5.

Tobacco Use Record

Time	Where am I / What am I doing / How am I feeling	Rating
6:00	*drinking coffee, just woke up*	5
6:30	*second cup of coffee*	4
7:00	*after breakfast*	3
7:30	*driving to work*	3
8:00	*parking lot, last one before work*	1
9:30	*break time*	4
9:35	*break time*	1
12:00	*leaving work for lunch*	4
12:30	*after lunch*	3
12:55	*parking lot, before going back to work*	1
2:00	*frustrated, took early break*	5
2:05	*frustrated*	2
3:30	*break*	3
5:00	*leaving work and driving home*	3
5:30	*fight with spouse, angry*	5
6:00	*after dinner*	2
7:00	*relaxing, watching TV*	3
8:00	*relaxing, watching TV*	3
9:30	*same*	3
11:00	*before bed*	3

A "1" is a low or no craving cigarette you don't physically need. You can take it or leave it. I call this a "movie" cigarette. You arrive at the movies early and smoke one. Not because you need it since you just smoked one in the car on the way to the theater, but you know you won't be able to smoke while sitting through a two hour movie.

A "5" is your strongest craving that can feel like, "*I'm going to die or go crazy if I don't smoke*". Often the first one in the morning, or when you have been unable to smoke for several hours, is a "5".

Don't wait until the end of the day to write down the specifics. Even if you remember every cigarette, it is almost impossible to go back and remember the intensity of the craving, which is the most important part of this activity; learning what triggers your "4's" and "5's" are linked with.

You will naturally cut down on the amount you smoke by rating your cravings because you will find "1's" and "2's" are easy ones to avoid. You won't smoke these because you have made smoking a conscious choice instead of an automatic reaction. You won't miss these cigarettes. When smokers cut down on their smoking, it is always the "4's" and "5's" which they keep and find the most difficult to stop from smoking.

Knowing where your weaknesses are ("4's" and "5's"), allows you time to prepare a strong defense. Strong cravings are often a downfall so it is helpful to give additional thought about how to avoid smoking when faced with these triggers.

Discover Your Obstacles to Success

Often smokers resist seeking help because, *"I've heard it all before."* Yet you can't know what you don't know. If you don't know what the problem is, you can't find a solution. Both the reasons why you smoke and the tools you use can be different than any other smoker.

Some obstacles to your success: physical dependency on nicotine, your unique beliefs about why you smoke and your specific fears about quitting.

Nicotine Dependence: Understand the physical effects nicotine has on your brain.

Nicotine is a natural substance found in the leaf of the tobacco plant. It is both a stimulant and a depressant depending on the dose. It can be lethal at high doses but does not cause cancer. Nicotine is the drug which causes the addiction, but it is the other chemicals which cause the various smoking-related diseases (see page 137).

While nicotine can be absorbed through your skin and the oral mucosa in your mouth, inhalation through your lungs is the most efficient and rapid way for nicotine to reach your brain, faster than injecting a substance into your veins. It takes less than 10 seconds or about 10 heartbeats for nicotine to get from your lips to your brain. The tobacco companies have further manipulated nicotine into a more potent "freebase" form allowing nicotine to quickly cross the blood–brain barrier, the structure which protects your brain from chemical toxins and bacterial infections passing into your brain.

Your brains communication network includes receptors, located on nerve cells, where neurotransmitters (brain chemicals) fit into like a key into a lock. Nicotine fits into a very specific receptor, located in the reward center or pleasure pathway of your brain, unlocking a flood of dopamine which is the *"I feel good"* brain chemical. Your brain "likes" this flood of dopamine. As you build up a tolerance to nicotine, your brain makes more of these specific receptors in order to have more dopamine circulating in your brain.

But your brain isn't used to this dramatic increase in dopamine and down regulates the amount. It is as if you are listening to music that is too loud, so you put ear plugs in to muffle the sound. Once you stop smoking, it can take time for your brain to adjust to a normal but lesser amount of dopamine (the music has been lowered to normal but you haven't taken the ear plugs out yet). This may be the cause of depression when quitting.

This increase in receptors and the dulling of excess dopamine is what makes the brain of a smoker structurally different than the brain of a non-smoker. This can happen by smoking as few as 100 cigarettes and is the start of a nicotine addiction. This does not mean that after 100 cigarettes you become a daily smoker, only that nicotine has already changed your brain structure, especially if you have started smoking as an adolescent, while your brain is still developing.

These changes may be permanent and may condition your brain to be more susceptible to other chemical addictions. This is why smoking has been called a "gateway drug". Nicotine is often the first substance used and it primes the brain for addiction to the next drug used. It doesn't mean that smoking will cause you to use another drug, only that if you do, you are more likely to become physically addicted compared to a non-smoker because an addiction pathway already exists in your brain.

The "*I feel good*" sensation doesn't last long. As nicotine leaves the receptors, cravings and withdrawal symptoms start as a reminder to refill the receptors with nicotine by smoking. A craving is just your brain shouting, *"Where's my nicotine?"*

The half-life or the time it takes nicotine to totally leave your body is quick, about three to five days. Many mistakenly think that once your body no longer has any nicotine in it that the withdrawals are over too. But this lack of nicotine in your body is what causes the intense withdrawals and cravings, which is your brain now *screaming* for nicotine. This continues until your brain receptors calm down and go dormant, which can take days, weeks or months.

Nicotine also hijacks the survival instinct part of your brain, the place where fear and compulsion come from. This is why a craving can often feel like, *"I'm going to die or go crazy if I don't smoke"*. These are your "4's" and "5's" from your Tobacco Use Record (see page 32). This part of your brain constantly scans, analyzes and interprets your environment looking for danger. It is a carryover from ancient survival skills telling you to play it safe and not make any changes because change is risky. Your instinct to survive is stronger than your willpower (the thinking part of your brain) which is why using willpower alone is a poor plan.

Unlike other addictive substances, nicotine is not a recreational drug used to get intoxicated but you need a certain amount of nicotine just to feel normal. Throughout the day you unconsciously self-regulate the amount of nicotine in your body to get your daily fix to feel normal by unconsciously adjusting how often you smoke and how deeply you inhale. This keeps the amount of nicotine in your blood system within your comfort zone, to avoid both nicotine withdrawals and overdose.

When you wake up in the morning, the amount is low, so you smoke several cigarettes to reach your comfort zone. If you smoke too much you will start feeling symptoms of nicotine overdose. If you don't smoke enough or go for several hours without smoking and have too little nicotine in your body, you start going through nicotine withdrawal. At night during sleep, the level falls again.

Nicotine Blood Levels throughout the Day

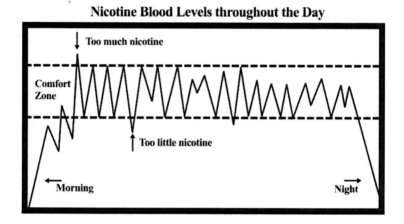

When you consciously try to limit the number of daily cigarettes smoked, you unconsciously compensate by smoking more intensely and/or deeply to stay in your comfort zone. If you want to cut back, substitute a fast acting nicotine medication for a cigarette, such as the gum, lozenge, inhaler or spray. You will reduce the amount smoked but because your nicotine blood level will be in your comfort zone, you won't compensate.

Activity: Take the Nicotine Dependency Test (see Appendix A on page 133).

Assess your physical dependency to nicotine and decide if you will use cessation medication(s) to ease your nicotine withdrawal symptoms.

Cessation medications can help any smoker through physical withdrawals so a low score does not mean that medications won't help you, but the higher your score, the more likely you are physically addicted and will have a harder time quitting without medication. Not every quitter needs medication, yet some smokers will find it impossible to quit without it.

Whether you should use cessation medications to control your withdrawal symptoms depends on several factors:

- How do you feel when you can't smoke for several hours? If you don't know, do a test by not smoking until noon one day and notice how you feel. Do you feel like, *"I'm going to die or go crazy if I don't smoke."*? Are you crawling up the wall or are you just uncomfortable? What is the longest period of time you have not smoked? If you have never been able to quit for more than a few hours or days, or find it almost unbearable to not smoke, medications will help relieve the physical withdrawals.

- Have you been addicted to alcohol or other substances? If yes, you may have a genetic predisposition to addiction. If you are sober now, you can use the same principles you used to abstain from your other addiction and apply them to nicotine.

- Have you been diagnosed with a mental illness? Individuals with depression, anxiety, schizophrenia or Post Traumatic Stress Disorder (PTSD) smoke more than the general population and may be self-medicating with nicotine, which may interfere with the efficacy of prescription medications for these disorders (see Appendix F on page 155).

Regardless of your score, all of these situations may indicate a greater physical nicotine dependency. It is important that you seek advice from a qualified medical professional who deals with nicotine dependency.

Reasons why cessation medications don't work. If you have used a cessation medication before and it "didn't work", identify the reason:

- Not having strong enough motivation. If you really don't want to quit, medications will not increase your motivation. If you relapse it is easier to say the medication did not work instead of admitting that you were not ready to quit. Medications are not a substitution for strong desire.

- Not understanding that there is more to quitting than just getting through the physical withdrawals. Medications only deal with the physical part of smoking; there is also a behavioral part. They can't be expected to take the place of learning how to live life as a non-smoker. For example: using medications won't help you deal with stress more effectively, they won't replace the feeling of having a cigarette with your coffee or having something in your hand.

- Expecting too much. Medications take the edge off of cravings and withdrawal symptoms. You still may have some symptoms but they should not be overwhelming. All cessation medications do is calm down the survival instinct part of your brain which then allows the thinking part of your brain (willpower) to take over and resist smoking. It moves a "4" or "5" craving to a "2" or "3" (see page 32).

- Not giving the medication a chance. Believing that using a nicotine replacement product is the same as getting nicotine from smoking, and by using it you will still be addicted to nicotine. Freebasing nicotine by inhalation gives a higher dose and is faster than any of the nicotine medications. None will give you the same jolt of nicotine or as fast an effect as you get from a cigarette. Medications are slower acting and need to be taken in advance, before a strong craving hits.

- Not using enough medication. Since the delivery system is not as potent or as fast as smoking, make sure you use enough of the product. There is no reason to be uncomfortable. If you are heavily addicted or have used one cessation medication unsuccessfully before, ask your doctor about trying combination therapy.

- Assuming if one medication did not work, the others won't either. Not every medication is appropriate for every smoker. Work with your doctor or pharmacist to help you decide which medication or combination is best for you. I have never met anyone who has used all seven FDA approved medications or combination of medications who was unsuccessful.

- Product is used incorrectly. Read the package insert to make sure you are using the product correctly. For example, don't wait for a craving to come up before reaching for the gum or a lozenge. Take them consistently throughout the day to ward off strong cravings. Your pharmacist can be a good source of information if the package insert is confusing.

- Not using them long enough. Often a smoker will think, *"I'm doing really well, I don't need to use a medication any longer."* But the reason they are doing so well is because they are using the medication to feel normal and are not experiencing extreme withdrawals. Think of how many years you have smoked. It is unrealistic to think that in a short period of time you will let go of your smoking behaviors, learn how to handle the social aspects and how to deal with stress. Don't stop the medications too soon and risk relapsing because you have not dealt fully with these other aspects. Just like when you learned to ride a bike, you needed training wheels until you developed basic riding skills to avoid crashing. Think of nicotine medication the same way; keep your training wheels on until you have the ability and skills to avoid crashing (relapsing).

- Thinking or being told that "cold turkey" is the most common and best way to quit. Don't let this belief get in your way of getting the help you need. Ex-smokers, who relapsed many times before finally being successful, may have learned how to deal with withdrawals without medications and will tell you that they don't work, but don't let their experience dictate what is best for you.

- Mistaking side-effects of cessation medications for withdrawal symptoms, nicotine or caffeine overdose and discontinuing treatment. Know the symptoms of nicotine withdrawal. If you are experiencing any of them, you may not be getting enough medication. If you are a heavy coffee drinker you may need to adjust the amount of caffeine consumed. Smoking interferes with the absorption of caffeine and it may feel like you are getting a double dose of caffeine after you quit. For any unexplained physical symptoms, talk with your healthcare provider:

  o Withdrawal symptoms: irritability, frustration, anger, anxiety, depression or feeling sad, difficulty concentrating, restlessness, decreased heart rate, hunger or an increase in appetite, inability to fall or stay asleep. Increase your dosage to relieve these symptoms or add another medication for combination therapy.

  o Nicotine overdose symptoms: Do you recall your very first cigarette? That is what nicotine overdose feels like: cold sweats, headache, dizziness, nausea or abdominal pain, vomiting, diarrhea, excess saliva, disturbed hearing and vision, muscle tremors, mental confusion and reduced oxygen to your skin. Reduce the amount of nicotine medication you are using.

  o Caffeine overdose symptoms: insomnia, nervousness, restlessness, irritability, stomach upset, fast heartbeat and muscle tremors.

o See Appendix D on page 141 for side-effects from medications which can be managed. Instead of worrying about the short term side effects of medications, think of the long term effects from smoking that you will be avoiding.

Activity: Decide how you will handle nicotine withdrawals.

Talk to your healthcare provider and decide if using medication is an appropriate treatment for you. See page 141 for an overview of FDA approved medications.

If you decide you would rather go a holistic route and avoid medications, then use the suggestions in Step Two (see page 70) and in Step Three (see page 86).

Beliefs: Discover your underlying beliefs about why you continue to smoke. Smokers usually start smoking for the pleasure they get from the flood of dopamine but continue to avoid the stress of the physical withdrawals.

Activity: Answer the following: *"I smoke because . . .*

. . . it relaxes me."

. . . it makes me feel good and I enjoy smoking."

. . . it gives me a 'high'."

. . . it's a reward after I finish a project."

. . . it's my only enjoyment in life."

. . . smoking's cool."

. . . smoking is my best friend."

These are all examples of **positive reinforcement**. The underlying belief is that you get so much enjoyment from smoking that nothing will ever give you as much pleasure as smoking does. You don't have to stop enjoying smoking, but to be successful and not relapse, you need something that is more important to you than a cigarette.

Smoking is really diminishing the good aspects of your life so instead, reframe your thinking to what smoking is depriving you of: good health, control over your life, better breathing. Stay focused on what you are getting by "Becoming Smoke-Free": freedom, more money, better health and more quality time with your family.

Smokers continue to believe they are receiving positive benefits from smoking, but they really continue smoking to avoid the negative effects of withdrawal.

Examples of **avoiding negative consequences**:

"I smoke because . . .

. . . it relieves my stress and helps me concentrate."

. . . it helps me deal with frustration and anger."

. . . I can't start the day without one."

. . . I'm addicted and can't live without my cigarettes."

. . . it stops me from being mean and keeps my emotions in check."

. . . I don't want to gain weight."

Once you stop smoking the amount of nicotine in your system drops, your stress level increases and your ability to concentrate decreases. You become irritable, angry and frustrated. Smoking a cigarette at this time will appear to enhance your ability to handle stress and concentrate better, yet all smoking has done is relieve your nicotine withdrawal symptoms.

The underlying belief is that smoking is the only option to release stress, help with negative emotions and relieve withdrawal symptoms. It is not the loss of pleasure but the avoidance of pain that keeps you hooked. Smoking is not the solution but the cause of these problems. Once the initial withdrawals have subsided, former smokers actually report less stress and negative emotions than when they smoked.

Which do you relate to more: the positive reinforcement or avoiding the negative consequences? There is a gender difference in that men often smoke for pleasure and women often smoke to help with negative emotions. For some it is a combination of both, but how you answer predominately, regardless of gender, can influence a choice in medications:

- If you smoke more for pleasure, ask your doctor about Chantix™, which blocks these sensations.
- If you smoke more to avoid negative emotions and withdrawals, ask your doctor about nicotine replacement therapy and/or Bupropion, which help relieve negative symptoms and weight gain.

Fear: Often our beliefs are stated as a "fear", which is just a belief that something "bad" will happen or you will lose something valuable. There is a feeling of dread, uneasiness and vulnerability.

Fear takes away your power for change and keeps you stuck right where you are. Taking action in the face of fear takes courage because fear exposes your vulnerabilities. Often the fear is the belief that you don't have what it takes physically, mentally and emotionally to endure the quitting process. Fear can also be a lack of confidence because you don't know how to cope without smoking (*therefore something bad will happen*) which just indicates new skills need to be learned.

Fear of Loss of Approval. Many smokers start smoking during their teen years to enhance their image—maybe appearing older, more sophisticated or as rebellious. Questions about your self-image can arise when smoking becomes too attached to your identity, such as:

"Will I be a different person once I stop smoking?"

"If smoking is cool, will I be 'not cool' if I stop smoking?"

"I won't know who I am if I'm not a smoker."

Smoking becomes so much of a smoker's persona that sometimes the fear is a loss of identity. Change is risky because you don't know who you will be on the other side of that change especially if you started as a teen and have never been an adult who doesn't smoke.

Fear of Loss of Control. There can be fear that when you quit, you will have no control over yourself or your actions; especially if when you quit before, you experienced severe withdrawals or gained a lot of weight.

Fear of Loss of Enjoyment. Quitting can feel like losing one of life's ultimate pleasures or your best friend. They have been there through the good times and the bad. They never talk back but have always given you exactly what you wanted. Quitting can be as traumatic as going through a divorce, learning to live life alone instead of with your cigarettes.

Activity: Uncover your underlying fears.

What are your fears about quitting? Spend some time thinking about your answers to the following questions before writing your answers in your notebook. See how your answers change over time.

- Is smoking a part of your self-image that was created when you started smoking? Are you a different person now and willing to let go of an outdated self-image?

- Are you scared that if you quit you will change? That you don't know what kind of person you will be and you may not like yourself as a non-smoker? Or that others may not like you; that you might become unlovable and be judged as unworthy by those closest to you if you change?

- While going through the quitting process, are you afraid you won't be able to control your actions or certain parts of your life if you quit? Are you concerned you won't know how to handle strong emotions and stress without smoking? Do you fear the loss of approval from others due to your behavior from nicotine withdrawal?

- Are you anxious that you will become a "reformed" smoker and your relationship with other family and friends who smoke will change? Or that your smoking friends will ignore, or abandon you?

- Are you worried you will never experience pleasure or enjoyment as a non-smoker, or believe that you can only have fun if you smoke? Do you feel you might be left out or deprived if you don't smoke?

- Are you more afraid of being called a "failure" for trying and not succeeding, than of continuing to be a smoker?

- Are you petrified you will gain weight and are fearful of what others will think of you and/or how you see yourself?

Use your answers to finish the following sentence:

"I smoke because I am afraid when I quit . . .

. . . I will gain weight."

. . . I will suffer pain when I quit."

. . . I won't be able to have fun anymore if I don't smoke."

. . . I won't know what to do when I have an intense craving. I won't be able to manage the withdrawals."

. . . I will fail again."

. . . I won't know who I am because I've always been a smoker."

Activity: Releasing fear meditation.

Sit in a quiet place, slow down your breathing. Breathe in for five seconds, exhale for five seconds. Repeat this breathing cycle as you let go of all thought. Relax as much as possible as you feel the tension leave your body by concentrating on your breath.

Imagine you are floating in the clouds. You are able to look down at your life like looking down at a road. You can see where you currently are, where you have been and where you are going.

See a situation in the past where you were also fearful or lacked the skills you needed to accomplish something. You overcame that fear and learned new skills. See that situation in your present life and notice the fear is gone. All you feel is a sense of accomplishment for overcoming your fear or lack of skill. Notice how good you feel.

Now imagine you are looking at your life one month from your Quit Date. There is no more fear of quitting. You are living your life as a non-smoker, feeling happy and pleased with your decision, feeling pride in your accomplishment. You see yourself having learned new skills to fill in where your cigarettes used to be. You see that you overcame your fear and successfully broke any connection to your fear of quitting. Those fears are gone, just like the fears you experienced in the previous situation you overcame. Notice how good you feel.

Reframe Your Obstacles to Success

Once you uncover the obstacles standing in your way, you need to reframe and/or change your limiting beliefs and fears. See page 115 for more information on reframing.

Activity: Make two lists, "Benefits of Smoking" and "Consequences of Quitting".

Your beliefs (see page 43) about the positive aspects of smoking are your "Benefits of Smoking" (*carrots*). Your fears (see page 45) are your "Consequences of Quitting" (*sticks*).

Carrots motivate you to continue your behavior but with smoking, the beliefs you have about the benefits, are not true. Smoking does not help your stress, make you happier or give you a better life, and when you really think about it, you actually don't enjoy smoking. You don't enjoy the taste, the smell, the cost, the burn holes, the health effects. Your only real enjoyment is the addiction. You may have been telling yourself these beliefs for so long that you believe them, but they are not true. Challenge every belief you have about smoking and realize it is time to let go of any false or out dated beliefs.

Benefits of Smoking	Consequences of Quitting
1. No withdrawals	1. Nicotine withdrawal
2. Don't have to change anything	2. Going to have to make changes
3. Handles my stress	3. Need new ways to handle stress
4. No change in weight	4. I might gain weight
5. No cravings	5. Strong cravings
6. I'm happier	6. I might be a jerk for a few days
7. No loss of smoking buddies	7. I might need new friends
8. No depression or anxiety	8. Depression and anxiety
9. It fills time	9. I need new activities
10. I enjoy smoking	10. I'll need to learn to enjoy life without cigarettes
11. My self-image stays the same a smoker	11. I need to figure out who I am as a non smoker

You need to reframe your beliefs about your "Benefits of Smoking" into your "Consequences of Quitting" — which show up as fears and obstacles (turn your *carrots into sticks*). Normally sticks are used to deny or avoid quitting. Your unwillingness to confront these issues are the reasons why you haven't stopped yet or have relapsed in the past. See page 15 about reframing.

It is natural to resist reframing this way because carrots are attractive and sticks are unwanted. Deal with your fears as an opportunity to learn more about your relationship to your cigarettes and what you need to learn to let go of that connection.

> *"On the other side of fear, lies freedom."*
> Marilyn Ferguson

Activity: Reframe each of your beliefs and fears to what you need to learn to be successful at "Becoming Smoke-Free".

When you finished the sentence, *"I smoke because . . ."* there is an accompanying unconscious and unspoken belief or fear that you will never find anything to take the place of your cigarette. You use this as a reason why you cannot quit. What beliefs and fears do you need to reframe so your thoughts work for you instead of against you?

"I smoke because it relaxes me (and I am afraid I will never find anything that gives me the same relaxation as a cigarette, therefore I can't quit)."

Reframe as: *"I smoke because it relaxes me and to be successful at quitting I need to learn how to relax without a cigarette."*

"I smoke because it relieves my stress (and I am afraid I will never find anything to relieve my stress, therefore I can't quit)."

Reframe as: *"I smoke because it relieves my stress, so I need to learn new ways of dealing with my stress to become smoke-free."*

"I smoke for something to do with my hands (and I am afraid I will never find something to do with my hands, therefore I can't quit)."

Reframe as: *"I smoke because it gives me something to do with my hands, so to be successful I need to find something else to occupy my hands."*

"I smoke because I enjoy it (and I am afraid I will never enjoy anything ever again, therefore I can't quit)."

Reframe as: *"I smoke because I enjoy it, so I need to learn how to enjoy life without smoking."*

"I smoke because I've tried before and failed (and I am afraid I will fail again, therefore I can't quit)."

Reframe as: *"I smoke because I am afraid I will fail, so I need to learn how to create a plan so I can be successful."*

"I smoke because I don't want to gain weight (and I am afraid that nothing will stop me from gaining, therefore I can't quit)."

Reframe as: *"I smoke because I am afraid I will gain weight, so I need to learn what I can do to avoid gaining weight to be successful."*

"I smoke because being a smoker is who I am (and I don't know who I am if I don't smoke therefor I can't quit)."

Reframe as: *"I smoke because being a smoker is who I am, so I will need to learn how to change my self-image to be successful."*

Don't always believe what you think. Decide your beliefs and fears are just something you tell yourself over and over again and may not be true. Instead, confront your fears about quitting and dispute your beliefs about any questionable benefits you assume you get from smoking. Dare to change your interpretation and perception of your beliefs and fears by learning the A-B-C-D Method described in Step Four (see page 118).

"In order to succeed, we must first believe that we can."
Nikos Kazantzakis

Commitment. Believe change is possible. Watch when you say, *"I'll try"*, or *"I can't . . . (quit smoking, deal with stress without my cigarette, etc.)"* Often *"I can't"* means either, *"I don't want to"* or, *"I'm not willing to do the necessary work"*. *"I'll try"* denotes a lack of a commitment

A commitment is the discipline to carry out a project, in spite of any obstacles and long after the mood has left you. It means that change is not a matter of *if* you will quit but *when* you will quit. It is a willingness to step outside your comfort zone and do whatever it takes to be successful.

Can you remember a situation when you were going to "try" to do something? Now think of a situation where you were totally committed and you amazed yourself? Notice how the outcomes differ.

"I'm going to try to quit smoking" is not a commitment but a vague statement. Instead, state what you will do and the time frame: *"I'm going to spend 10 minutes each day working on my Plan."*

Don't concentrate on what you are unwilling to do; there are always alternatives. Figure out what you are willing to do and make a contract with yourself to do it. View this time as a learning opportunity, not an obstacle.

Any time you feel apprehensive or panic-stricken about quitting, don't push yourself. Fear is about a future event.

Focus on the present moment and what you can do right now, not on what might happen in the future.

To break the gridlock when you are paralyzed with fear, take a baby step and do something easy. You will gain confidence by doing something simple until you feel comfortable to take another baby step, then another. It is normal to feel awkward when trying something new. Don't use fear as an excuse to procrastinate and do nothing.

Be a realistic optimist and be willing to give up unrealistic expectations about what quitting should look like, or how long it will take. Remember this is a process and not a one-time event. If you wanted to lose weight, you wouldn't think that all it takes to drop weight is to wake up tomorrow and you would have dropped 10 pounds. You did not become a smoker overnight and it is unrealistic to think you can quit overnight.

Be open to new information instead of clinging to old beliefs which may no longer fit your perception of yourself. Decide to trust yourself that you will be okay physically, mentally and emotionally as a former smoker. Decide you have the ability to learn the skills you need to be successful and the resources you need will be available. Decide you can think about the quitting process in a different, more positive way and take the anxiety out of it.

Listen to what you tell yourself about quitting and your relationship with your cigarettes. Write down in your notebook any random thoughts that enter your mind. This is your subconscious telling you what issues you need to work on. Don't ignore that small voice inside.

If you are not ready to make a commitment to be smoke-free, and are still working on your desire, instead of saying, "*I have to quit*" or "*I should quit*" and reframe it to "*I'm working on building my desire.*"

Quitting may be one of the hardest things you ever accomplish in life and it's easy to become discouraged but quitting is also one of the most rewarding achievements. Doing the activities and answering the questions in this book might not be what you want to do or it may feel uncomfortable, but make the commitment because you know you need to do it to be successful.

Activity: Compare and contrast lists. Compare the new lists you made on page 49: "Benefits of Smoking" and "Consequences of Quitting" to the two lists you made earlier on page 9: "Benefits of Becoming Smoke-Free" and "Consequences of Continuing to Smoke".

When you think about smoking, your brain will want to continue your behavior because change is risky so your thoughts will automatically veer towards your perceived "Benefits of Smoking" (lower right corner) and will deny any "Consequences of Continuing to Smoke" (upper left corner) and will try to avoid your "Consequences of Quitting" (lower left corner).

To be successful your reasons to "Becoming Smoke-Free" (upper left corner) have to be more important than your "Benefits of Smoking" (lower left corner) *and* have to be worth going through the "Consequences of Quitting" (lower right corner).

Instead of obsessing about the benefits or pleasures of smoking, concentrate on your reasons to be smoke-free.

Make what you value by "Being Smoke-Free" more important than the reasons why you smoke (see page 8).

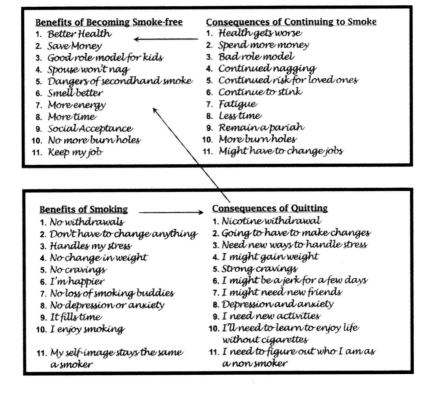

Recognize that the reason why you continue to smoke and/or relapse is because you have not successfully confronted your unrealistic beliefs about why you continue to smoke and have not resolved your fears about quitting.

Examine your thoughts, beliefs and fears, and reframe them to your advantage. The arrows on the chart are where you want to lead your thoughts:

- Reframe the enjoyment of smoking to be a "Consequence of Quitting".
- Reframe the "Consequences of Quitting" as hurdles to be overcome for your true goal of "Becoming Smoke-Free". Write each of these obstacles down in your notebook and think of strategies to deal with each one. In Step Two you will learn how to figure out what tools will help you overcome these problems.
- Reframe the negative "Consequences of Continuing to Smoke" as positive "Benefits of Being Smoke-Free".

Notice that the "Benefits of Becoming Smoke-Free" are all long-term and the "Benefits of Smoking" are short-term. By smoking one cigarette you stop withdrawals immediately and you feel better but it can take some time before you feel noticeably better after "Becoming Smoke-Free". You won't save a lot of money by not smoking one cigarette or improve your health by not smoking one cigarette. This is how smokers fall into the trap of thinking they can smoke "just one", which is a delay tactic and prevents you from getting what is truly important to you. Make the decision which carrots are more important to you: the "Benefits of Becoming Smoke-Free" or the "Benefits of Smoking".

Realize you cannot continue to delude yourself about continuing to smoke *and* being able to avoid the negative "Consequences of Smoking". Smokers think it will always happen to the other guy and not to them. Realize you are the other guy.

Challenge for Step One:

This compare and contrast chart is the real work for Step One: Build your motivation by having important personal reasons to "Become Smoke-Free". Remove the obstacles to reaching that goal which are your idealistic beliefs about your deceptive "Benefits of Smoking" and your seemingly overpowering fears about the "Consequences of Quitting".

All the Activities in this Step are to give you an insight into your relationship with tobacco. The first step to any solution includes having a complete understanding of the problem, resolving your ambivalence about letting go of your past bond with smoking, and embracing your smoke-free future.

"Just remember, you can do anything you set your mind to, but it takes action, perseverance and facing your fears."
Gillian Anderson

"Do or do not. There is no try."
Yoda

Step Two: Create Your Action Plan

- Set a Quit Date
- Make a Personalized Action Plan
- Countdown to Quit Day
- Challenge for Step Two

> *"Smokers don't plan to fail, they fail to plan."*
> Author Unknown

In Step One you added some missing pieces to your smoking puzzle by learning about your personal relationship to smoking. You are working on building your motivation as well as reframing your beliefs and fears. Now you will use that information to create your personalized Action Plan to quit. Having a personal Plan is essential to be successful and remain smoke-free. Smokers often underestimate the value of having a Plan and being prepared. Instead they go "cold turkey" and rely on willpower. Confidence and success come by practicing and refining your Plan before you quit.

Think back to when you learned to drive. At first, it felt awkward but with practice, driving became automatic. Now imagine your doctor said you had to quit driving because it caused cancer or heart disease. You would immediately go into a panic: *"How do I get to work in the morning, or go to the grocery store? How can I live without my car?"* With some planning, you can manage: You could walk, ride a bike, take a bus, subway, metro, plane or train, skateboard, or ask friends and family for a lift. There are many different modes of transportation which can be used to avoid driving a car. But in an emergency, you still know how to drive. Your brain will forever have a memory imprint of how to drive a car.

The same thing happens with smoking. At first it was awkward, then it became automatic. If you feel you have to quit smoking before you have a Plan in place, you immediately start to panic: *"How do I have my coffee without smoking? How do I drive without a cigarette? How do I handle stress without smoking?"*

Just like it would take some time to figure out alternatives to driving your car, it will take some time to figure out alternatives to your smoking behavior. The way to be successful is to make a Plan for the different situations and then practice.

> *"The secret to change is to focus all of your energy not on fighting the old, but on building the new."*
> Socrates

Activity: Set a Quit Date.

Select a Quit Date preferably within two to four weeks, and work up to it. Don't choose a date in the distant future, such as a year from next Sunday, you will procrastinate and not follow through.

Mark the date on your calendar. Make a commitment to work on your personalized Plan every day until then so you are fully prepared. One way to almost guarantee failure is to set a date, do nothing to prepare, and expect to rely on willpower alone. Would you wake up tomorrow vowing to not drive and not have a plan on how to get to work?

Decide whether a weekday or the weekend is better for you. If your workplace is smoke-free and you don't smoke at work, choose a work day. If you don't smoke around your family, plan a family day or quit on the weekend.

Choose a day which will be easiest to refrain from smoking or that has a special importance attached:

- Your birthday or the birthday of a child or spouse.

- If you have lost a loved one to smoking, choose their birthday and quit as a tribute to them.

- Mother's or Father's Day in honor of a parent.

- The anniversary of your sobriety from other substances.

- Valentine's Day is a good day to show you love yourself.

Don't choose a day where you will be tempted to smoke:

- Social events you must attend such as birthdays, anniversaries, Super-bowl parties, reunions, and other occasions where you would be tempted.

- When you will be socializing with your smoking friends, especially if alcohol is involved.

- When you have plans to visit your smoking buddy or when your in-laws, who smoke, will be visiting.

- When you will be under added stress due to work or other obligations.

Ideally you want to have at least a two-week time period where you will be able to fully concentrate on going through the quitting process so you will have the best possible chance to stop and avoid relapsing.

If it is normal for you to have ongoing stress in your life, don't use this as an excuse to continue smoking and not set a Quit Date. There is no better time than the present if you don't see an end to continuous pressure. Read the section on Becoming Stress Hardy in Step Four (see page 114). Reframe your situation knowing that quitting will lessen your stress.

Spontaneous Quit. If you are not ready to set a date, continue working on your Plan and eventually you will feel comfortable picking a Quit Date or you will wake up one morning and decide today is the day you no longer smoke. Often the timing of *when* to quit is spontaneous, like a light switch suddenly turned on. If you have been diligently working on your Plan, you will know when you are ready because you are well prepared.

Activity: Figure out how much time you spend smoking.

Five minutes per cigarette times twenty cigarettes equals 100 minutes, or about an hour and a half each day spent smoking. That is over 22 days in one year. Allow for a longer time if you have to walk a great distance to a smoking area.

Give up two "1" or "2" rated cigarettes a day (about 10 minutes). Use the time you would have spent smoking them to work on developing your Action Plan.

"A goal without a plan is just a wish."
Antoine de Saint-Exupery

Make a Personalized Action Plan

Use what you learned in Step One about your unique relationship with cigarettes to create a personalized Action Plan which addresses your particular reasons for smoking, habits, beliefs and fears.

Break your automatic "habit" cigarettes before you quit. The conditioning of your brain to expect nicotine has become linked to almost anything in your environment and will now trigger a craving: sitting down in your favorite chair or at the computer, smelling coffee or getting into your car. Give yourself the opportunity to break your knee-jerk behavior while your brain is still getting nicotine.

Activity: Make a Smoking Corner and Smoke by the Clock.

Set up a place to smoke which is away from all household activities — someplace you don't normally go, and only smoke there. It could be the side of the house, by the garbage cans, in a corner of the garage or down the street at the neighbors' garbage can. Don't make it someplace you enjoy going to, rather someplace you don't like and don't normally spend much time there.

If you already smoke outside, for example on your patio or porch, find someplace new. After you quit smoking, you want to be able to go to your patio without it triggering a craving to smoke. Change the place where you used to smoke to a new relaxation corner where no smoking is allowed. Practice your relaxation techniques there and/or use this area to work on your Action Plan.

Smoke by the Clock. Schedule your smoking. Don't smoke whenever you want to, instead let the clock dictate when you smoke. Choose a time schedule so you smoke often enough to avoid having strong cravings or withdrawals:

- 10 cigarettes a day equals 1 every two hours.
- 20 cigarettes a day equals 1 cigarette every hour.
- 40 cigarettes a day equals 1 every half hour.

Once you decide on how often you will smoke, only smoke at those times. For example: If you choose to smoke one cigarette an hour and you wake up at 6 am, smoke your first cigarette at that time, then again at 7 am, 8 am, 9 am, etc. and every hour for the rest of the day. Don't smoke at any other time. If you have physical withdrawals, decrease the time interval between cigarettes or use a short acting nicotine medication, but don't smoke when you want to, only when the clock dictates.

If you don't feel the need to smoke when it is your time to smoke, you don't have to, but acknowledge you cannot have another cigarette until it is your next "time to smoke". Don't try to cut down—the purpose is to learn new behaviors while breaking your old associations and not go through nicotine withdrawals at the same time.

When it is your "time to smoke", go to your Smoking Corner, stand (unless you have a physical challenge) and smoke. In your Smoking Corner, don't do anything else except smoke. Don't take your coffee with you. Don't take your cell phone. Don't listen to your iPod. Don't leave a window open and watch TV. Don't talk to others. The purpose is not to multi-task when you smoke but to give yourself time to be conscious of what you are doing. By separating your smoking behavior from your other behaviors, you are "breaking your habit".

After you have smoked a cigarette, go back into the house and go about your normal activities. Have your cup of coffee, watch television, or sit at the computer. See how it feels to be doing this activity without smoking. It might feel weird, but this is normal. Remind yourself that this strange feeling is just a thought about smoking and not a physical craving. This is the time to practice the alternative behaviors you have been thinking of trying which will become the basis for your Action Plan.

Stop smoking in your car. If you are driving when it is your "time to smoke", pull over to a safe area and get out of your car to smoke. Leave your cigarettes in the trunk.

Don't smoke with other people. If your work place has a designated smoking area, stand off to a corner by yourself. Don't socialize with your fellow smokers while you smoke. It's OK to talk with them but not while you have a cigarette in your hand.

If you are at a social event, don't smoke with others but go off to a secluded area to attempt to stay with the spirit of having a Smoking Corner. When at a friends house, don't join them in smoking but let them smoke and you go outside by yourself when you want to smoke.

Activity: Track your triggers.

Since you are breaking your "habits" by having a Smoking Corner and Smoking by the Clock, mark down in your notebook each time you don't smoke with one of your common triggers and by the 30th time, your connection will be broken. But if during this time, you slip and smoke with that trigger, your brain lights up and says *"Ah ha, you can't fool me, if I wait long enough I'll get some nicotine."* It still connects that activity with smoking, so it is important to not smoke with that trigger until it is "extinguished" or you need to start counting all over again.

Since your brain has thousands of memory imprints of different "habit" cigarettes, it is not unusual to have a thought come "out of the blue" even if you have been quit for a long time. Remember, it is just a thought and not a true physical craving. See page 123 for more information about "out of the blue" triggers.

Activity: Create an Action Plan.

Develop and practice different strategies, techniques and tools to deal with your smoking triggers.

On the left side of a piece of paper, list your common triggers for each part of the day (morning, afternoon, evening) from your Tobacco Use Record (see page 32); be sure to include the "4's" and "5's". You may need several different strategies to deal with these strong cravings.

My Action Plan

My common triggers:	What I can do instead of smoking:
Mornings:	
Coffee	Switch to tea, add flavoring
After breakfast	Take a shower, brush my teeth
Driving to work	Take sips of water, hold a straw
Afternoons:	
Break at work	Read a book, sit with non-smokers
After lunch	Eat a mint, play a game on phone
Frustrating phone call	Squeeze a stress ball, deep breathe
Evenings:	
Driving home	Eat raisins one at a time
Fight with spouse	Go for a 5 minute walk
After dinner	Clear table and wash dishes
Watching TV	Sit in a different chair or room

In Step One, you were asked to identify the different connections you have to smoking and to think about alternative behaviors. List those ideas on the right hand side under, "*What I can do instead of smoking*". These are the tools you can start practicing to see what works for you.

You were also asked in Step One to reframe your limiting beliefs and fears into what skills or tools you need to be successful at quitting smoking. Include ideas to deal with those issues and list them on the right hand side under, "What I can do instead of smoking".

Once completed, this is your Action Pan to follow during the first days of your quitting process. New situations may arise which you haven't prepared for; try what has worked in other situations, and revise your Plan as needed. Don't rely on will-power alone; remember it is not stronger than your survival instinct.

> *"If the only tool you have is a hammer,*
> *then every problem looks like a nail."*
> Abraham Maslow

Toolbox Approach: If you were going to build a table, you would need several different tools: a hammer, saw, level, measuring tape and more. It might be impossible to build a table if you only had a hammer to use.

To quit smoking, don't rely on just one tool but develop a variety of tools. You may need many different tools in your "quit smoking toolbox" where each can be used in many situations: the tool you use when driving might be sunflower seeds, the tool for after a meal might be taking a walk and the tool for your morning coffee is to sit in a different chair. Cessation medications are a tool for nicotine withdrawals.

Sometimes you will need a specific tool for a specific trigger. Practice alternative behaviors several times to see what works best for you. Don't give up after one try. Don't feel discouraged if you try something and it doesn't work. Every method will work for some smokers; no method works for everyone. The challenge is to keep trying out alternatives until you find out what does work for you.

For any trigger there are only two choices: You can change your behavior and/or you can change your thinking. "Habit" cigarettes often need a change in behavior (do something different). "Emotional" cigarettes need a change in thinking (change how you think about smoking from it being a helping friend to how it is impairing your life). Your job is to personalize the behavior change and your thoughts.

If you have quit before, what techniques worked for you then? Ask former smokers what worked for them. For additional ideas, read Appendix G: The Seven "D's" on page 158.

Countdown to Quit Day

Everyone has rituals in daily life. Think of how your day is thrown off when, for some reason, your morning ritual is disrupted. Perhaps you ran out of coffee or the newspaper didn't show up. It throws your routine off, sometimes for the whole day. A cigarette has fit into your morning ritual at the same time and place every day. Often that first cigarette is a hard one to give up because it is both a physical craving and a habit connected to the same time, activity and place each morning. Plan for that disruption in your morning ritual and replace it with something else.

Now realize you have 20 rituals a day which are no longer there. Cigarettes are connected to your life in so many different ways. It is normal to feel like something is missing and/or to grieve the loss of an old friend.

The better prepared you are, the easier it is to quit and not relapse. Runners train for months to be in the best possible shape before a marathon; without preparation they might only make it half way. The longer you practice Smoking by the Clock in your Smoking Corner and developing your Action Plan before your Quit Date, the more prepared you will be to make it in the long run. Many of your habits will be broken, your rituals adjusted and you will find it easier than the times you have quit when you were not prepared. You will feel confident in your ability to carry out your Plan because you have practiced and made it unique to your behavior.

Activity: Decide on different strategies to prepare you physically and mentally, change your behavior, manage your environment and find support.

Get Ready Physically:

- Speak with your physician if you have any health problems before making any changes in your routine or starting an exercise program.

- Drink plenty of fluids to flush your system. Water is best. Supplement with fruit juices containing vitamin C but limit them if weight gain is a concern. Drink enough until the color of your urine is clear.

- Heavy caffeine users risk a caffeine overdose (see page 42). Cut back on your total caffeine intake from coffee, tea and energy drinks. Coffee is often a trigger to smoke, but can cause headaches if abruptly stopped.

- Smoking generates an acidic condition. To aid in detoxification and withdrawals, start eating an alkaline diet consisting of fresh fruits and vegetables, preferably raw. Stock up on crunchy low-fat foods such as carrots, celery, radishes, broccoli, bell peppers, apples, pears, cinnamon sticks, sugarless candy, unbuttered popcorn, rice cakes and non-sugar cereal. Use these to satisfy your hand-to-mouth motion and oral fixation.

- Take a multi-vitamin with extra vitamin C and vitamin B's. Nicotine may reduce blood levels of vitamin B-12, and smokers need three times the amount of vitamin C as a non-smoker.

- Get plenty of rest. Your body is going through trauma and needs the restorative nature of sleep. Try to sleep enough each night that you don't need an alarm to wake you. Don't take on extra responsibilities at this time which will add to your stress.

- Exercise helps with unwanted weight gain and stress. Walk briskly for 20 minutes each day. This can be two separate ten-minute sessions. Take a walk in place of your morning cigarette or on your break at work when you used to smoke.

- Start the habit of deep breathing. It can have the same calming effect as smoking a cigarette by slowing down your heart rate. Breathe in through your nose for five seconds, expanding your abdomen, then breathe out through your mouth for five seconds. With each breathing cycle, increase the length of time you are exhaling by one second until you are exhaling twice as long (ten seconds) as you are inhaling (five seconds):
    - Breathe in for five seconds, out for five.
    - Breathe in for five seconds, out for six.
    - Breathe in for five seconds, out for seven.
    - Breathe in for five seconds, out for eight.
    - Breathe in for five seconds, out for nine.
    - Breathe in for five seconds, out for ten.

- Avoid alcohol for several weeks. Alcohol impairs your judgment. If you won't stop drinking alcohol, you may want to look at your reasons why and consider talking to a specialist to see if alcohol is a problem also. If you are a heavy drinker, talk to your doctor before stopping drinking which can cause debilitating withdrawals. Heavy drinking is defined by the Centers for Disease Control and Prevention as having more than 15 drinks in a week if you are a man and more than 8 drinks in a week if you are a woman.

- Make a survival kit containing gum, cinnamon or vegetable sticks, cheerios or other non-sugar cereal, plastic straws and other items to chew on or twist. Get a water bottle, taking sips to mimic hand-to-mouth motions. Carry a book or Kindle, a crossword puzzle or have games on your phone for moments of boredom. Get a stress ball.

- If you are using cessation medication(s), purchase your over-the-counter (OTC) medications or have your prescription filled before your Quit Date. Start substituting a nicotine replacement product such as the gum, lozenge or inhaler for a cigarette as a way to taper down and eventually switch from smoking to using a cessation medication.

Get Ready Mentally:

- Continue to read your Reasons to Quit Card before you light up. Find new "Benefits to Become Smoke-Free".

- As often as possible throughout the day, repeat positive thoughts: *"I love the thought of being smoke-free because . . ."* Then think of one of your personal benefits of quitting: *"I love how much money I'm going to save."* If positive statements are not motivating, think of an image which scares you, or something you want to avoid. With every puff, think, *"Another breath of cancer."* Or, *"I'm sucking on the tailpipe of a car."* Or imagine a tiny gas chamber over your head. Or image your pack is twenty little terrorists trying to kill you.

- Visualize yourself in situations where you would normally smoke—what would you do as a non-smoker? For example, when at work, what can you do on your break instead of smoking? What are non-smokers doing? Watch what non-smokers do with their hands, see how they handle stress without smoking. Ask former smokers what has helped them stay tobacco-free.

- Make a "pre-commitment". Find something you hate and decide that if you slip and smoke even one cigarette, you will have to do this action. For example, if you slip you must write a large check and donate it to a political or social organization that you hate. Make that deal with yourself and don't give yourself a way out. Any time a craving comes up, think about how it would feel to have to write that check—is one cigarette really worth it?

- Quitting can feel like getting a divorce. It is normal to grieve this loss. Writing a goodbye letter to your cigarettes helps provide therapeutic closure to this toxic relationship. Tell them how you met, what they have meant to you, how they have both helped and hurt you, and also why you need to end this relationship:

Dear Marlboro 100's, I've loved you since I was 14 when I was a shy teenager and smoking gave me confidence. Now

30 years later, it's time to say goodbye, I want to be smoke-free because . . ."

Change Behaviors and Manage Your Environment:

- Make smoking inconvenient, unpleasant and awkward. Change brands of tobacco to something you don't like. Switch from regular to menthol, or menthol to regular. If you start to like the new cigarettes, switch brands again. Buy only one pack at a time instead of cartons. Smoke with your opposite hand.

- Keep your cigarettes as far away as possible. Don't carry them with you but leave them in your Smoking Corner, in another room or in the trunk of your car. Make it so that you have to get up and go get them when you want to smoke.

- Don't smoke where you normally smoke such as in your favorite chair. Only smoke in your Smoking Corner and only when it is your "time to smoke". Break the associations you have with your normal routine.

- If you are not Smoking by the Clock, practice delaying having a cigarette. Wait five or ten minutes after the urge comes up before you light up.

- Continue refining your Action Plan. Notice any new triggers and think about new coping strategies. By recording your smoking behavior on your Tobacco Use Record so that smoking becomes a conscious choice, more of your sporadic smoking connections are revealed.

- Get rid of all tobacco equipment such as ashtrays, lighters, and matches. If you take the ashtray out of your car, keep it for when you want to sell the car, but don't use this as an excuse to litter the street with butts.

- Collect your cigarette butts in a glass jar, fill it with water and use it as an ashtray in your Smoking Corner. Use this as a visual reminder of what the cigarettes are doing to the inside of your body. Walk your yard, pick up all thrown butts and put them in the jar.

- Make it part of your Action Plan to avoid going to the gas station or grocery store where you normally buy cigarettes. Go to a different location where the visual cues are different than the store/gas station you are used to. Either stock up your groceries for the week or get someone else to go for you or with you.

- Clean your house to get rid of the cigarette residue. Have your clothes cleaned to remove the smoke smell. Detail your car. Open your butt jar and take a whiff to remind yourself of the stench of stale smoke you want to rid your house, car and clothes of.

- Find all hidden packs or loose cigarettes. Search purses, jackets, under car seats, in your cars glove-box, the freezer; anywhere cigarettes might be hiding. Don't stash a pack "just in case" or to prove you are stronger than the urge to smoke one. Before you go to bed, have a funeral, then "Crush and Flush" all remaining cigarettes. Don't just wet them down and throw them in the trash because you might be tempted to dig them out and dry them off with a hair dryer. If you can't bear to toss your unsmoked cigarettes, stay up all night to finish the last of your pack if you must but don't have any cigarettes in the house the morning of your Quit Date. If you can't bear to be without a pack, realize that cigarettes are as close as an all-night convenience store and they don't need to be in your home where the temptation might be too great to resist. Having to drive to pick up a pack gives you time for to the craving to pass.

Find Support. Often smokers want to go it alone when quitting, especially if they have relapsed before because they don't want to let anyone down. But your journey will be easier by having strong support from family and friends, professional support which gives you guidance and education, and by keeping your guard up for saboteurs.

Social Support. Talk to people you see every day such as family, friends and co-workers before your Quit Date. Ask for their help, get them on your side. Be open with them about working on your Action Plan. You never know where good advice and support can come from. Most people do want you to succeed.

If you have quit before, tell your loved ones why this time is different. Read them parts of this book to reinforce this different way of thinking. Tell them exactly the kind of support you need, whether you want constant attention or want to be left alone or somewhere in between. Be specific about how they can be supportive.

Those who have never smoked have absolutely no idea how hard it is to quit or how they can help. Expect them to not understand. They may say the wrong thing because they don't know any better. Support can also be what they should not say. Remind them of statements they have made in the past which were not helpful. Tell them what they could have said that would have been helpful.

Don't tell them that you are quitting or have quit, only that you are working on a plan and need their assistance. If you say you are quitting and you are seen smoking, you may be confronted with, *"I thought you were quitting?"* and feel the need to defend yourself.

By saying, *"I am working on my Plan"*, you reframe the situation which explains how a great deal of work needs to be done before you finally put down your last cigarette. Tell them about your Smoking Corner, Smoking by the Clock and any other tools you are using.

Ask your supporters to help you celebrate your milestones in the future: one day, one week, one month, three months, six months and one year. Ask them to make a big deal out of it, because this is a big deal.

After your Quit Date, instead of feeling apologetic if you slip, reframe the situation so a lapse is a *"practice run that needs refinement"*. Tell them the challenge you are working on and how they can help. Also ask them to congratulate you even if you slip for a great *"practice run"* instead expressing disappointment over a lapse. Ask them to remind you that a slip or relapse is just a stepping stone towards your final success.

Decide how you will act around other tobacco users. Talk to the smokers in your life BEFORE you quit. Once you quit, you are no longer "one of us" (a smoker) but "one of them" (obnoxious ex-smoker). Even if you don't change, their perception of you could.

With your friends and family who smoke, make a "deal" with them: promise to not nag them about quitting if they will support your quitting effort. Ask them to not give you a cigarette after your Quit Date, even if you beg them for one. Tell them if they do give you a cigarette, the "deal" is off and you can nag them about quitting. Let them use this "deal" as the reason to NOT give you a cigarette and as an incentive for you to not ask in the first place. If you don't make a "deal", then plan a response if you are offered a cigarette. Tell them that you might have to avoid them WHILE they are smoking and you will rejoin them once the cigarette is out. Don't sit with them when they smoke even if it is not an overwhelming temptation. When you smell smoke, your brain's desire for nicotine can trick you into believing you can have "just one" to be social. If you are at their home, ask yourself why you put yourself into temptation's way.

If you live with another smoker, talk about boundaries before you quit. The conversation will vary depending on whether it is a spouse, significant other, adult child, parent or roommate. Agree on which areas of shared living space where smoking will be allowed and where it will not. See if they will agree to only smoke in your Smoking Corner also (just not at the same time as you). If not, ask the smoker to not leave dirty ashtrays and open packs out because of your attraction to them.

They may complain that it is not fair for you to ask them to make any changes. If they refuse to be supportive, then you must be overly prepared and cautious. You can quit but your journey will be more difficult. Decide that no matter what, their behavior is not going to influence your quest for freedom from nicotine. Strength comes from your preparation, commitment and desire.

The smokers in your life may surprise you. As they notice how strong you are while they are weak in their nicotine addiction, they may decide to quit too and ask you for help.

Closet smokers. Some smokers hide their behavior because they don't want their friends and family to nag them. They don't want to hear the disappointment, the anguish, the frustration in their loved ones voice. Closet smokers feel a range of emotions from failure, shame and guilt to indignation and self-righteousness. The problem is when a closet smoker wants to quit, it's hard to ask for help for something you've hidden from everyone. It doesn't mean you don't want to quit but it's hard to admit to your use of tobacco. If you are a closet smoker, asking for help may be difficult for you but fessing up can lighten your burden.

"You're only as sick as your secrets."
Alcoholics Anonymous

Professional Support. Make an appointment with your doctor, nurse, dentist or other healthcare professional:

- Talk to a Tobacco Treatment Specialist. Call 1-800-Quit-Net for free telephone counseling. Surf the web for free information (see Appendix B on page 135 for a list of resources). Call your local county health department for local resources.

- Take the Nicotine Dependence Test (see page 133) and discuss the results with your doctor. Ask if a FDA approved cessation medication is appropriate for your physical condition as well as your mental health history, including any eating disorders, depression and anxiety. Tell your doctor about any current or history of alcohol and other substance use.

- Make sure your doctor knows all the medications you are taking including any over-the-counter ones because they may work differently after you quit smoking; also include heavy caffeine use. The dosage may need to be adjusted after you stop smoking since nicotine interferes with the efficacy of some medications, see page 155 for a partial list.

- Read the product safety information and package insert for the medication and ask your doctor or pharmacist about any concerns you have about side effects. Many can be effectively managed and need not be a reason to stop the medication.

- Make an appointment with your dentist to have your teeth cleaned and have an oral examination.

Saboteurs. Sometimes loved ones can have the best intentions of offering support, but instead sabotage your progress by nagging, shaming or blaming. You feel like they are trying to hit you over the head with the biggest *stick* they can find.

You know the personalities of the various people in your life. Decide who may make verbal sabotage attacks. Either avoid them as much as possible, learn to tune them out, or assert yourself and tell them how hurtful their comments are.

If you experience extreme withdrawal symptoms of anger, and/or irritability, some people may suggest you go back to smoking. Show them your Nicotine Withdrawal Card (see page 91) and explain nicotine withdrawal symptoms are normal and temporary. Tell them you are asking them to be an angel while you may act like the devil. Your symptoms won't last forever, but the damaging effects of smoking can last a lifetime.

Beware of close friends and family who smoke and may miss your smoking times together. They may want their "old smoking buddy" back and not honor your "deal". If you expect your smoking friends to be negative, talk about *your* reasons why it's important for *you* to be smoke-free or, blame your doctor, *"My doctor says I have to quit."* Then say that it may be too tempting to be around them when they smoke and your health is dependent on you quitting.

A former smoker can either be a great support person or a saboteur especially if they feel their way is the only way to be successful and criticize your method.

So beware when a former smoker says, *"I've tried EVERYTHING and nothing worked until I used (acupuncture, hypnosis, herbal tea, a Peruvian amulet) and you should try it too."* Their method may have value and be something you can add to your toolbox, but don't let them sway you away from the tools you feel you need to be successful. They had a lot of tools in their toolbox, not just the last one used.

Often a smoker will sabotage their quit attempt because their motivation is not strong enough. Be honest about how much you really want to be smoke-free versus how much you want to continue smoking.

Don't lie to yourself about how you feel or what you do. For example, purposely going to visit someone who smokes because you really just want to bum a cigarette. Resist the temptation to steal one from an open pack, thinking that no one will be the wiser. You are only hurting yourself by being less than honest.

Sabotaging yourself includes: lying to yourself, not taking care of your physical and emotional needs, knowingly going into tempting situations to see if you are strong enough to resist, making excuses — there are no longer any reasons to smoke, only excuses.

Activity: Make a list of support people with their phone numbers and people to avoid:

Think about the different people in your life. Who will be a good support person and who would likely be a saboteur?

Consider your family, both those you live with and extended family, close friends and casual acquaintances, co-workers, social groups, Facebook pals. Who is a former smoker who may be a good support person or who may have kept you at a distance because you smoke?

Find a "quit buddy", another smoker who is quitting, so you can give each other support. Find a sponsor by joining a Nicotine Anonymous group. If there is not one in your area, think about starting a chapter. Join BecomeAnEx.org or another online support group.

People to avoid: smokers who will tease or tempt you with a cigarette, someone who is not supportive and might undermine you whether or not they smoke, people who encourage you to go back to smoking or tell you that you will never make it.

Challenge for Step Two:

The mission for Step Two is to be prepared by taking action. Often it is not *what* you do that is important but that you are *willing* to do something that is important. All the Activities in this Step are to spur you on to not just think and read about quitting, but to show you the value of preparation by taking action which will increase your confidence.

"Knowing is not enough; we must apply.
Willing is not enough; we must do."
Johan Wolfgang Van Goethe

"Knowing what to do doesn't mean much unless you do it."
Author Unknown

"One important key to success is self-confidence. An important key to self-confidence is preparation."

Arthur Ashe

Step Three: Your First Smoke-Free Week

- What to Expect
- How Fast Your Body Heals
- Reminders for Your First Week
- Challenge for Step Three

What to Expect

Give yourself a pat on the back! Look how far you have come since you started this journey. Often smokers (and their family and friends) don't give themselves enough credit for the steps leading up to their first smoke-free day. The work done up to now is vital to your success.

Be a realistic optimist. Prepare to feel uncomfortable and be pleasantly surprised when it is easier than you thought because of your preparation and planning. How good you feel this week will depend on several factors:

- How strong is your motivation to "Become Smoke-Free"? See page 101 on motivation and short-term relapse.

- How well did you prepare? Did you take the time to write in a notebook and do the preparation work, or did you skim through the material? One advantage of having a quit buddy, sponsor or working with a Tobacco Treatment Specialist is accountability.

- If you practiced Smoking by the Clock in your Smoking Corner for any length of time, you will feel more comfortable because you will have broken many of your habits already. If you didn't, remember it will take three to four weeks or 30 consecutive actions to extinguish the automatic response of your "habit" cigarettes.

- What did you not do? This is your weak area. It is normal to do what is easiest instead of what is needed but harder to do. Did you prepare physically but not do anything about your behavior? Or did you not ask for the kind of support you need? Whatever area of preparation you neglected will be where you will have problems.

Activity: Recognize the physical withdrawal symptoms of nicotine and develop strategies for coping:

Strong cravings or urges to smoke: Nicotine is a powerful drug, but the craving will pass whether or not you smoke.

- Exercise, go for a walk. Distract yourself, call a support person. Use a fast-acting nicotine medication: gum, lozenge, inhaler or spray.

Depressed mood: Nicotine binds with receptors in the pleasure pathway or reward center of the brain. With nicotine withdrawal, some quitters may experience severe depression.

- Take time to enjoy pleasurable activities. Reward yourself for your hard work at quitting. Be kind to yourself and ease up on unrealistic expectations.
- Don't self-medicate with alcohol and/or other substances. Decrease your consumption of alcohol if you are using Chantix.
- Seek out professional help if depression is disrupting your work, home life or ability to get along with others.

Insomnia or sleep problems: Nicotine is a contradictory drug—both a stimulant and depressant. Withdrawing from it can also have contradictory effects: some cannot stay awake, some cannot go to sleep.

- Stop caffeine by early afternoon. Learn relaxation techniques. Listen to calming music, take a soothing bath. Use the deep breathing exercise on page 71. Ask your doctor about appropriate sleep hygiene ideas such as: Don't eat before going to bed. Don't watch TV in bed. If you can't sleep, get up and go to another room.

Fatigue: As a stimulant, you may feel tired or listless without nicotine.

- Take a cat-nap in the afternoon. Take a brisk short walk. Splash cold water on your face.

Anxiety, irritability, frustration and anger:

- Exercise, deep breathing and relaxation techniques will reduce these withdrawal symptoms.

Restlessness, difficulty concentrating:

- Take frequent breaks. Take a brisk walk. Allow extra time to complete your responsibilities.

Increased appetite or weight gain:

- Keep a survival kit with you packed with low fat, crunchy vegetables, gum, straws, toothpicks, cinnamon sticks. Drink water. Read the suggestions in Step Four: Avoid Weight Gain (see page 120).

Recovery Symptoms are not considered "withdrawals" but are other physical changes which happen when you stop smoking that you also need to be aware of:

Cold or flu symptoms: The first few days many feel sick.

- Stay in bed and drink plenty of water. Treat yourself lovingly like you do when you are physically ill.

Dry mouth, tender gums, mouth sores and/or tightness in the throat:

- Use teething gel. Suck on throat lozenges or hard candy, sip warm herbal tea.

Intestinal problems: Some have diarrhea and others are constipated.

- Drink more water and add high fiber foods to your diet.

Increased cough: Many quitters experience an increase in coughing. The hair-like cilia in the lungs, whose job is to clear out debris, are paralyzed from smoke and never get a chance to "clean up". They start working overtime when you quit smoking. It is not uncommon to cough more in the first month after you quit.

- Take an over-the-counter product such as Mucinex, suck on cough drops. If the coughing persists longer than four weeks, see your doctor. If you have smoked one pack for 30 years, or two packs for 15 years (each are considered a "30 pack-year" smoker) and are over the age of 55, ask your doctor if a <u>low-dose</u> spiral CT scan is an appropriate screening test for you.

Time distortion: Time seems to slow down. Your first day lasts FOREVER. The first week seems to last a month.

- Plan to keep busy this first week since you will have plenty of time on your hands. Increase doing activities you enjoy. Do projects you have put off because you haven't had the time: Spring clean the house, declutter the garage.

Dizziness, feeling light headed, headaches and confusion: A main component of smoke is carbon monoxide. When inhaled, this gas binds to your red blood cells faster than oxygen, depriving your body of the oxygen it needs. Your body compensates by increasing the number of red blood cells. Smokers are often told they have "thick" blood. When you quit smoking, extra oxygen is taken in by the higher number of red blood cells. It takes about three weeks for the body to adjust the number of red blood cells.

- Be careful when changing positions such as from lying down to standing up. Use handrails. Use caution when getting up from prolonged sitting or from bed.

- Some headaches are due to dehydration, so drink plenty of water and add a magnesium supplement.

- Give blood at the blood bank.

Tingling sensations or numbness in your fingers and toes: Smoking constricts your blood vessels. When you quit smoking, the blood flow increases and can cause sensations like when your foot "falls asleep".

- Be sure to be steady on your feet when standing. Massage the bottoms of your feet by rolling them over a tennis ball. Exercise your hands by clenching and unclenching your fists.

Improved complexion: As your blood vessels open up, color returns to your skin. The lack of oxygen to your skin from smoking is a major cause of wrinkles.

- Smile as your complexion improves and enjoy the compliments as others notice too.

Hypersensitivity to smells: You will be surprised at how other smokers stink once you have quit. You will wonder if you smelled the same way.

- Enjoy pleasant new aromas and avoid foul smells. Light scented candles, have flowers near or use an air deodorizer.

Caffeine overdose: Nicotine interferes with the absorption of caffeine by 50 percent. Once you stop smoking, the same amount of caffeine you are used to can cause a caffeine overdose (see page 42).

- Decrease your caffeine intake, including energy drinks, sodas and tea.

Reframe your withdrawal symptoms to "recovery symptoms", or *"My body is cleaning out the toxins."* Remember these physical symptoms are time limited and don't last forever, yet they are a major cause of relapse.

Stay in touch with your doctor. There is no need to be extremely uncomfortable. If you are not using a cessation medication, and you are having intense withdrawal symptoms, rethink your choice to not use medication. The use of a medication is for a short period of time while the damage from smoking can last your whole lifespan.

If you are using cessation medications, the dosages may need adjusting; increasing the dose if you continue to have withdrawal symptoms. The dosages of your regular meds may need adjusting too.

If you are having side effects from medications, often the dosages and/or the timing can be changed; such as taking them with food if you have nausea, or several hours before bedtime to reduce weird dreams and/or insomnia. For severe effects, switch to a different medication.

Activity: Make a Nicotine Withdrawal and Coping Strategies Card.

Make a card similar to your Reasons to Quit Card (see page 17), listing the physical nicotine withdrawal symptoms on one side and on the other side list The Seven "D's" (see page 158) and a couple of your personal ideas. Carry this card with you.

Nicotine Withdrawal and Coping Strategies Card

Side one   **Side two**

Remember: These are NORMAL Nicotine Withdrawal Symptoms:	Coping Strategies for Withdrawals:
Depression, restlessness, irritability, anxiousness, anger, having difficulty concentrating, sleep problems and increased appetite	Drink water, Deep breathing, Delay Do something else, Distract my thoughts Discuss with friends, Don't Smoke: NOPE, Not One Puff Ever!
These symptoms are most intense the first 2 weeks but may last several month	

Read your Card anytime you are experiencing a withdrawal symptom to remind yourself that what you are going through is *normal*. Then look at the back side for what you can do to get through it.

If a friend or family member mentions your behavior, show them your Card and inform them your behavior is typical. Ask for their help in getting through this phase and explain this will not last forever. However, if they mention noticing severe depression, aggression, suicide ideation or other abnormal behavior, call your doctor immediately.

How Fast Your Body Heals

Notice how much better you feel and remind yourself how fast your body is recovering. Watch the time add up after you quit and realize how your body is improving:

After 20 minutes:

- Your blood pressure and pulse rate drop to normal.
- The temperature of your hands and feet increases.

After 8 hours:

- The carbon monoxide level in your blood drops to normal while the oxygen level increases to normal.

After 24 to 72 hours:

- Your chance of a heart attack decreases.
- Your nerve endings start to grow again due to increased blood supply.
- Your bronchial tubes relax, making breathing easier. Your lung capacity increases.

After 1 to 2 weeks:

- A pregnant woman provides her fetus with nicotine-free blood.
- Your sense of taste and smell improves.
- Your skin color improves as the circulation to your skin improves.

After 1 month to 1 year:

- Your blood circulation improves, your hands and feet feel warmer.
- Your heartbeat will slow down and your blood pressure will drop.
- Coughing, wheezing, respiratory infections, bronchitis, sinus congestion, fatigue, shortness of breath—all decrease.
- The small hair-like cilia that clean out your lungs become more active, increasing ability to clear mucus, clean out your lungs and reduce risk of infection.
- Your overall energy level and stamina improves.
- At one year, your risk of heart disease is reduced by one half.

After 5 years:

- The lung cancer death rate for the average smoker (one pack a day) drops almost in half.
- Your risk of cancers of the mouth, throat, esophagus, pancreas and bladder drop by half.
- Your risk of a stroke, cervical cancer and cancer of the larynx (voice-box) is the same as a non-smoker.

After 10 years:

- The lung cancer death rate for the average smoker drops to almost the half rate of non-smokers. Precancerous cells are replaced.
- The rate of other cancers, such as those of the mouth, throat, esophagus, bladder, kidney and pancreas continues to decrease.

After 15 years:

- Your risk of heart disease and death rate are similar to that of a non-smoker.

Reminders for Your First Week

Decide you will do whatever it takes to avoid slipping. Be prepared to overcome any obstacles you meet. When tempted to smoke or have "just one", remember your "pre-commitment" and imagine if you slip how much you will hate having to write a large check to an organization you can't tolerate. Repeat to yourself, *"Smoking is no longer an option"* or *"I don't do that anymore"*.

- Carry your survival kit (see page 72) with you to keep your hands and mouth busy. Include your Nicotine Withdrawal Card and/or Action Plan. When a craving hits, you don't have to think about what is happening or what to do, it's all written down. Your Reasons to Quit Card should be with you too. Review it whenever a craving comes up. Remind yourself what is truly important—it's not the cigarette.

- Watch what you are putting into your mouth. It can be tempting to overeat and overindulge in sweets. See page 120 on avoiding weight gain.

- Calculate how much money you have saved (see page 10). Use this money to reward yourself for quitting for one day, one week and/or after avoiding a powerful craving. See page 21 for ideas for rewards.

- Figure out how many cigarettes you have not smoked in one week or how many puffs you have avoided (see page 30). Be proud of each and every one dodged.

- Continue to avoid situations where you might be tempted to smoke. If a craving seems overwhelming, reach out to a support person or your quit buddy.

- Avoid alcohol for several weeks. If you are unable or unwilling to stop drinking, you may want to consider that you have an alcohol dependency.

You always have a choice! It is important to not slip and smoke any cigarettes but since you are only human, slips do happen. Stop a slip when a craving first comes up. You always have two choices:

- You work through it and remain smoke-free, or

- You slip and smoke a cigarette.

If you choose to slip, again you have two choices:

- You resolve to remain smoke-free and learn from the slip, or

- You blame yourself, beat yourself up, feel guilty and smoke another cigarette.

If you choose to smoke another, your next two choices are:

- You renew your resolve to become smoke-free and start anew, or

- You relapse and become a smoker again. Realize you need to work on your motivation, make changes in your Action Plan and/or set another Quit Date when you're ready.

You can choose to see a slip as a failure or as a learning experience. You can choose to let the events of your life control you, or you can take control of your life. The choices you make are determined by who you think you are, and the benefits and expectations you bring to the situation.

Activity: Five steps to train your brain to think of smoking in a different way.

You need to recondition your brain to stop the automatic thoughts that nicotine has planted. It takes time. If you only change your behavior and not your thinking, you may relapse or turn to something else such as food.

Whenever a craving comes up, use these steps to change the way you think about smoking and having a craving. You can use these steps when you first quit and at any time in the future:

1. *"I'm having a desire to smoke right now."* Recognize you are having a desire to smoke. This is normal. The craving will go away whether or not you smoke. Just let it run its course.

2. *"I can smoke at any time, I'm not deprived."* Nobody is taking your cigarettes away from you. It is your choice. Remember what smoking is really depriving you of that is more important: your money, health, and freedom.

3. *"I'm a puff away from a pack a day."* It's easy to fall into the trap of having "just one". Don't kid yourself that your willpower is stronger than a nicotine addiction.

4. *"Right now I have a choice to make for myself. Either I give in to this temporary discomfort and go back to the constant misery of smoking, or I can accept this temporary discomfort and work through it for . . ."* (name one of your "Benefits of Becoming Smoke-Free").

5. *"At this moment, I willingly accept this temporary discomfort because I want . . ."* (then list your "Benefits of Becoming Smoke-Free"). Focus on your personal values that are truly important to you that smoking is depriving you of.

Challenge for Step Three:

DON'T SMOKE, no matter what. This is the time to use all the tools, techniques and strategies you have been practicing to avoid smoking. Revise your Action Plan as needed to overcome unexpected circumstances. Develop new tools as new situations arise. Don't tell yourself you are only going to have *"just one"* to get through a craving. Reintroducing nicotine into your brain does not help; it only sets you back.

"Surprise yourself every day with your own courage."
Denholm Elliott

"Do something today that your future self will be proud of."
Author Unknown

Step Four: Prevent Relapse

- Understand Relapse
- Long-Term Maintenance
- Develop an ICE Plan
- Challenge for Step Four

"Our greatest weakness lies in giving up. The most certain way to succeed is always to try just one more time."
Thomas Edison

The first part of your journey is to Stop Smoking. The second part is to Stay Quit by maintaining your nicotine abstinence. Staying smoke-free long-term is like walking down a road full of landmines. You have the best of intentions of staying smoke-free but then you step on a hidden landmine and boom – you have relapsed.

This section is going to tell you what will cause you to relapse and how to prevent it. Unfortunately, this is the part that most quitters ignore, which is why there is such a high relapse rate. About one third of all smokers try to quit each year and up to 95 percent will be smoking again within six months to a year.

It is normal for a smoker to make many serious quit attempts before they finally quit for good. Personally I had nine serious attempts each lasting at least three months but I also had countless tries some only lasting a few hours or days. Learn from my mistakes at relapsing and decide to make this your last time.

> *"It's easy to quit smoking, I've done it hundreds of times."*
> Mark Twain

Understand Relapse

If you wanted to drop weight, you need to be willing to change your food intake and increase your physical activity. This takes a commitment, making a Plan and taking action. Slowly over time the pounds come off.

If after six months you went to a birthday party where your favorite chocolate fudge cake was being served and this one time you are unable to resist treating yourself to an extra-large corner piece with lots of frosting, you would not gain back the pounds you lost (you would if you continued this way of eating, but not from one slip).

Now imagine if you are at same birthday party but instead of being tempted by the cake, the temptation is a cigarette. Social events are when you enjoyed smoking the most, everyone is celebrating, alcohol is involved and it doesn't feel the same without smoking. A friend is smoking your brand and offers you one. You slip, smoke it and the receptors in your brain get flooded with dopamine. Your brain seductively says, *"Don't tease me with one, I want the whole pack"*.

The dopamine makes you feel better, big red warning flags don't pop up to caution you of the landmine right in front of you and you give yourself permission to smoke another one. Within a few cigarettes, your brain expects to have the same level of nicotine it had been used to prior to quitting, and you will relapse to your previous level of smoking. It would be like eating "just one" slice of chocolate fudge cake and overnight gaining back all the weight you had lost in the previous six months. It will feel as if you had never quit. Many will get discouraged feeling all their hard work is for nothing and won't try to quit again for years. Don't let this be your experience.

Learn the difference between a slip and a relapse. A slip is an "oops"; "*Oops, I slipped and smoked one or two cigarettes*". It means you have something more to learn about being smoke-free. It indicates a situation came up where you justified saying "*yes*" or it overwhelmed your ability to say "*no*" (like being at that birthday party).

A slip doesn't need to turn into a relapse but a relapse always starts with a slip. Avoid thinking you have failed. Reframe the slip as a learning experience. What happened? What can you do instead when this situation comes up again? Recommit to "Becoming Smoke-Free".

Realize any slip could lead you straight back to smoking full-time. For some, a slip leads to a return of a consistent pattern of smoking, such as, "*I only smoke three a day, one after every meal*", or "*I only smoke when I drink*" which a smoker will rationalize as "*not so bad.*" But your brain is like a spoiled child throwing a tantrum until it gets what it wants which is for you to go back to smoking as many as you did before you quit. Once you have been a full-time smoker you will never be able to be a "social" smoker or be able to smoke "just one" now and then. You might know some people who are able to be a "social" smoker but they have never been addicted like you have been.

A slip or a relapse can happen at any time. The timing of when it happens provides a clue as to what issue needs to be addressed and added or changed in your Action Plan.

Short-term relapse usually occurs within the first 30 days, however it could be longer for those heavily addicted to nicotine. It is usually related to lack of motivation, nicotine withdrawals and/or "habit" cigarettes.

It is common for relapsers to blame their return to smoking on their method, such as cessation medications, instead of owning up to the fact that their motivation was lacking. It is only later when they quit for good that they will say that previous attempts didn't work because they really didn't want to quit. To be successful long-term means having compelling personal reasons to stay Smoke-Free and maintain your sobriety from nicotine.

Severe nicotine withdrawals are a common reason for relapsing. Some heavily addicted smokers can have prolonged withdrawals lasting up to six months, however the symptoms will fade out over time. The use of combination cessation medications can greatly relieve the physical withdrawals and cravings.

If you set up a Smoking Corner and "Smoked by the Clock" (see page 63), most of your habit cigarettes should be broken before your quit date (see page 31).

The following indications mean you have made it through the short-term relapse phase:

- The nicotine withdrawals have lessened or stopped. They no longer are overwhelming. You feel normal most of the time.

- You no longer crave one of your normal "habit" cigarettes.

- You realize you have gone all day without thinking about a cigarette.

- You forget how hard it was to quit. You might even say it was easy and you get complacent.

Long-term relapse occurs after you feel like a non-smoker most of the time. You have made great progress up to now; but keep conscientious. You are still at a high risk for a relapse. Research shows that the rate of relapse steadily drops through the first two years after quitting yet a nicotine addict will remain at risk for a relapse at any time for the rest of their life.

The reasons for a long-term relapse are different than the ones for a short-term relapse:

- A crisis situation triggers an intense craving which overwhelms your ability to cope, causing high levels of stress or negative emotions. Now when a smoker slips it is not because they have a "1" or "2" rated craving, it is because a "5" craving overpowers them.

- Parties or pleasant social events, positive feelings, or rewarding yourself.

- Weight gain.

- Consuming alcohol.

- Being around other smokers.

- Getting too cocky. You think you can control your smoking and only smoke when you want to. Don't get overconfident. You cannot control your smoking and smoke one or two when you want. Don't test yourself to see if you can resist temptation. I've had several clients quit for as long as twenty years, yet relapse after smoking just a few cigarettes.

"Your best teacher is your last mistake."
Ralph Nader

Activity: If you have relapsed before, was it a short-term or long-term relapse and what was the reason?

Instead of viewing a previous relapse as a failure, look at what you did learn from the experience. You picked up a couple of different tools. You were able to avoid some triggers. Look at how many cigarettes you were able to avoid! You also learned what did not work for you.

This is a time to be brutally honest with yourself. Is what actually happened different than what you have told yourself? Such as blaming your relapse on a medication not working when it was your motivation that waned or that you didn't have the tools to deal with extreme stress. To be successful you need to look at what didn't work the last time instead of doing the same thing over and over.

It can take several attempts before a smoker is successful. Often during the first couple of quit attempts, a smoker will figure out how to avoid a short-term relapse. They have learned how to ease withdrawals with or without medication, they have tools to deal with their habits and since they feel normal without smoking, they don't develop tools to deal with a long-term relapse. Once a smoker finally does quit for good, frequently they will give credit to the last "method" they used, instead of seeing the reason why they were finally successful was because of the accumulation of experience and knowledge from previous "failed" attempts.

"I have not failed.
I've just found 1000 ways that won't work."
Thomas A. Edison

Long-Term Maintenance

Emotional Triggers. After you quit, your emotions may be more intense, or you may be more aware of your feelings. Smoking helps regulate emotions through the release of dopamine; positive emotions are enhanced and negative emotions are lessened. Smoking offers the illusion of being able to go through life with the least amount of pain and greatest amount of pleasure.

There are four ways of dealing with emotional needs: suppress, escape, express and release. Smoking is a form of suppressing or "stuffing" feelings. When intense or strong feelings arose, often a cigarette was the first thing you reached for to satisfy your emotional needs in the past. If you started smoking as a teen, you have not had practice dealing with strong emotions without smoking. Don't switch your method of suppressing or escaping by self-medicating with other substances or destructive behaviors including: alcohol, illicit drugs, over-the-counter or prescription medications, gambling, sex and computer use. They don't fulfill your emotional needs or remove the conditions but only add to your difficulties. Instead develop new healthy solutions:

- When angry, the emotional need is to release or let it out: Scream. Smack a pillow. Hit the gym and work it out. Write a letter to the person you are angry with, keep writing until all your anger is gone then burn the letter.

- Loneliness is a need for emotional intimacy: Express it by calling a close friend. Speak to a counselor. Volunteer to help others in need. Get a pet.

- When feeling sad, express your sadness: Cry if needed. Share your troubles with an understanding friend. Seek counseling from a professional if your depression affects your ability to enjoy life.

- Expression is the emotional need for happiness: For a period of time after quitting, it may feel like you aren't able to be happy and celebrate without a cigarette. It feels like something is missing which is the flood of a dopamine. Its effect has been dulled (like using ear plugs) and your body doesn't recognize a normal amount as being enough (instead of the music being too loud, you are unable to hear normal tones). As the receptors in your brain calm down and recover (the ear plugs are removed), you will discover you can enjoy situations without smoking. Until then work on changing your attitude by using the suggestions on reframing (see page 115).

- When fearful or afraid, the need is to release it and feel safe: Smoking gives a false sense of security. It does nothing to help a threatening situation. In fearful situations, smoking does not calm your nerves; it increases stress hormones. In severe situations, such as battle, smoking may play a role in the development of Post-Traumatic Stress Disorder (PTSD). See page 45 for more information on fear.

- When your feelings are hurt, comfort is sought: Express it by journaling about your feelings or talking to a friend.

- When bored, the emotional need is for the expression of doing worthwhile activities: Once you quit smoking, you will have a lot of time on your hands. Develop new interests, take a class or start a new hobby. Volunteer your time to help those less fortunate. Find some passion project that can fill your time; something new and exciting.

- Guilt is about living in the past and wishing you had done something different or the feeling you did something "wrong": Festering guilt can cause depression, anxiety, anger, resentment and remorse. It can cause self-dislike, hatred and can destroy your self-esteem. The emotional release for guilt is to express forgiveness for yourself for your past actions. It means learning from your behavior, taking responsibility for your conduct, making a commitment to live in the present and not do it again. If your actions affected someone else, decide if an apology is appropriate. Often guilt is felt when nothing "wrong" was done.

Decide to be assertive and stand up for your rights instead of feeling guilty.

- Two common emotions felt by smokers are guilt and shame: The normal cycle of a smoker trying to become smoke-free is: Stop, relapse, quit again, relapse again. This can bring a sense of guilt: *"I'm doing something wrong"*, or shame: *"There is something wrong with me that I can't quit"*. Neither is true. It's not your fault. There is nothing wrong with you except to realize how powerful a drug nicotine is, how it has controlled you, why you need gripping desire and a solid Action Plan.

- Feelings of depravation will disappear over time. Quitting smoking can feel like losing a best friend and can leave a void in your life. Cigarettes have been there through everything, as a way to cope, for comfort, to celebrate or commiserate, and to help you feel safe. It is normal to mourn this loss but you won't not miss your cigarettes forever—instead they will be replaced with an appreciation for all your positive benefits of "Being Smoke-Free". Write a goodbye letter as closure to that toxic relationship (see page 73).

Handle Stress without Smoking. The human stress reaction is a holdover from caveman days with the "Fight, Flight or Freeze" response which describes how our nervous system reacts to stress.

Your autonomic nervous system (ANS) has two parts: sympathetic and parasympathetic, which control the same organs but in opposite ways, like a yin/yang relationship. When faced with danger, your body readies to either run away, stand and fight, or hide. Once the threat is gone, the other part of your ANS takes over and the body relaxes. In the modern world, our perception of "danger" can put the nervous system into a semi-permanent state of "Fight, Flight or Freeze" with a constant release of stress hormones which affect you physically, mentally and emotionally.

Activity: Understand how many different ways stress may affect you. Make a list of which of the symptoms on this graphic which may apply to you.

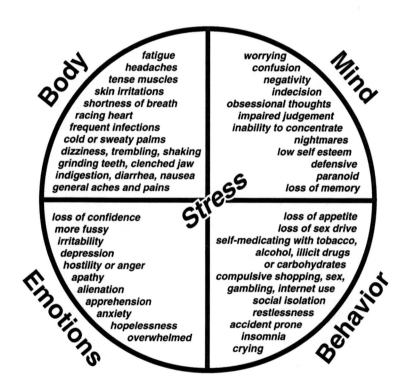

Stress is a major cause of relapse because smokers lack other stress reducing options. Smoking has been an easy, low-effort coping behavior that you have used to deal with stress and strong emotions. Smoking provides temporary relief from the physical stress of nicotine withdrawal, which is the reason why smokers mistakenly believe that nicotine is an effective strategy for stress. It feels like it helps to decrease negative feelings such as tension, anxiety and anger, yet realize you are self-medicating and not actually dealing with your problems.

Anything can be stressful. What is stressful for one person, may not be for someone else; it is how you perceive the event and react that makes it stressful, not the actual event. For example, traffic seems to be a stressful event for many, yet to others, it's not a bother at all.

To be stressful the situation also has to exceed your ability to cope. Think of stress as adding water to a glass. Your coping skills are like a release valve so your glass doesn't get too full. There are varying degrees of stress such as having a flat tire which is inconvenient and would be like adding a few drops of water to your glass. Having a major car accident which wrecks your car and puts you in the hospital would like having your glass flooded. But even small irritations and inconveniences can add up, drip by drip until your glass is overflowing if you don't have adequate coping strategies to relieve some of the pressure. As stress builds this can lead to various physical maladies, emotional and mental trauma.

After becoming smoke-free, when a cigarette is no longer a coping option, minor incidences of stress will be magnified yet you will probably be able to handle the small stuff. It is when an unexpected situation arises that exceeds your ability to cope and endangers your well-being, that a cigarette feels mighty tempting if other resources are not available.

Your behavior is how you relieve stress. If negative behaviors, such as smoking, are used to suppress or escape, it increases your stress, not relieve it. You need to develop new healthy ways of coping with stress. The solution will depend on your level of stress and the type of relief needed; whether it is physical or emotional relief.

Activity: Decide how you can relieve your physical symptoms of stress, how you can cope emotionally and mentally, and resolve to not act out behaviorally.

- Learn how to deep breathe: Stress can cause people to take shallower breaths which decreases your focus and concentration. You can relieve the tension in your body by inhaling deeply and allowing your lungs to take in as much oxygen as possible. Think of filling a glass with water; it fills from the bottom up. It should be the same way with your lungs. Place your hands on your abdomen right above your bellybutton. Inhale deeply and slowly for five seconds through your nose and feel your stomach expand. Exhale for five seconds through your mouth and feel your stomach contract. This is one example of a breathing exercise, another type is described on page 71, where your inhalation time is increased.

- Learn progressive muscle relaxation: Systematically tense, then relax the different muscle groups of your body. Start with your dominant hand and forearm, then move to your upper arm, your non-dominant hand and forearm, upper arm, forehead, upper cheeks and nose, lower face, neck, chest, shoulders and upper back, abdomen, dominant upper leg, calf, foot, non-dominant upper leg, calf, foot. For each muscle group, hold the tightened muscle for 10 seconds before releasing; notice the difference in how the muscle feels from being tense to being relaxed.

- Pamper yourself: Do things you find relaxing. Take a bubble bath. Go for a long walk outdoors. Enjoy nature and reflect on the peacefulness of a flower or tree. Have lunch with a friend. Stay home and read. Get your spouse to take the children and have an afternoon for yourself. Get a massage. Let your batteries recharge. Make room in your life for more fun activities. Pet your dog or cat.

- Exercise to relieve tension: Set up a program you enjoy. Find an exercise buddy or walk the dog.

- Take a yoga, meditation or tai chi class which can help physically as well as calm your mind.

- Release your emotions: Cry; a good cry can be a healthy way to release tension. Laugh; laughter can release "feel good" chemicals in the brain.

- Listen to something that makes you feel good: Relaxation tapes, classical or soothing music.

- Daydream or visualize about a calm peaceful place in nature where you have been before: Clear your mind, close your eyes and imagine you are there. It is restful; maybe lying on the beach, sitting by a lake or hiking in the woods. Try to remember what sounds you heard. Seagulls, birds or the wind? Do you feel the sun on your skin, or are you under the shade of a tree or have sand in your toes? What do you smell? Flowers, the ocean, the freshness after a rain? A few minutes reliving a peaceful scene can give you a mental break as well as relax your body and relieve your tension.

- Share your stress: It helps to talk with a friend about your concerns and worries. A different perspective is often helpful. Seek support from friends or family members. If stress is interfering in everyday activities, consider talking to a licensed therapist or find a support group.

- Learn to say *"NO"* to excessive demands: Know your limits. Turn off your phone and computer. Allow yourself to schedule "me" time; if you are asked if you have a commitment, say *"yes"*. You don't need to say it's *"me"* time or share that it is a commitment to take care of yourself, just say that you are busy.

- Ask yourself, *"Does it really matter to me?"* Be willing to let go of unimportant issues. Don't sweat the small stuff and remember, it is all small stuff.

- Go with the flow and learn to be more flexible. Avoid or alter the cause of your stress. Be proactive, expand your horizons, and think creatively or outside the box. Learn and practice the Serenity Prayer:

  > *God grant me the serenity*
  > *To accept the things I cannot change*
  > *Courage to change the things I can*
  > *And wisdom to know the difference*

- Learn what you have control over and what you don't have control over. If a situation cannot be changed at this time and is beyond your control, don't fight it.

Learn to accept it for what it is now, until such time that you can change it.

o You have direct control over problems with your behavior. You can change your habits.

o You only have indirect control when you have problems with the behavior of others. You can change how you interact.

o You have no control over the past or other situational realities. You can change the way that you see it. See page 115 on reframing.

• Take a time management class: Get organized, clean up the clutter. Spend 15 minutes doing one thing you have been procrastinating about, you may not finish but you might find the task easier than you thought. Pursue obtainable goals: Make a list of what you *will* do this week, not what you think you *should* do, but what you are *capable* of finishing. Learn to prioritize your commitments; not everything is an emergency. Learn to live in the moment and make a decision as to what is the most important thing you can do right now; don't try to multi-task, but concentrate on one item.

• Remember to "HALT" whenever you are: Hungry, Angry (Alcohol, Anxiety), Lonely, and/or Tired; common triggers which are neglected and cause undesired consequences.

Decide to Become Stress-Hardy. Improve your ability to handle stress by improving your physical and mental state through nutrition, exercise, relaxation, and amplifying positive attitudes and emotions. The most stressful times, such as a death in the family, a catastrophic illness or accident, job loss or divorce, can happen at any time and the impact can have damaging effects (see page 109). Decide to improve your physical and mental health to withstand difficult times. Quitting smoking is the best lifestyle change you can make. Decide to improve the other areas of your life as well, either now or after you have been quit for a while.

- *"What is the one change I can make in my food intake to make it more nutritious?"*
- *"What can I do to exercise more?"*
- *"What can I do to relax instead of smoking?"*
- *"How can I think in a more positive manner?"*

"If you can't change your fate, you can change your attitude."
Amy Tan

Reframing or Changing Your Attitude. Several times you have been asked to reframe your words to something that will support your goal of "Becoming Smoke-Free" instead of hindering your desire, and to alter your beliefs and fears about quitting into a positive attitude.

Reframing is a psychological term meaning making a conscious shift in your perspective or mindset to a healthier, more optimistic viewpoint—a change in attitude. Many smokers have a negative, pessimistic view of quitting, which constricts thinking and triggers a stress response. When confronted with quitting, smokers will defend their "right" to smoke (fight), they will avoid the people encouraging them to quit (flight) or will deny or negate that smoking is causing a problem (freeze). None of these responses are constructive.

Reframing is not a "Pollyanna" style of thinking that ignores or denies negative emotions or situations, but shifts a person out of a stress response into an action mode and promotes personal growth. Obsessing or ruminating on the negative prevents a person from moving forward and finding a solution.

An open attitude towards difficulties in life, such as quitting smoking, can help you generate human strengths as you develop new resources to deal with the adversity of quitting: resilience, creativity, persistence, problem solving, confidence, ingenuity, critical thinking, courage and self-control.

> *"Optimism is the faith that leads to achievement."*
> Helen Keller

Activity: Develop tools to change your attitude.

Experiencing positive emotions (not just the absence of negative emotions) can improve your coping responses to stress. Positive and negative emotions are not mutually exclusive; even in the depths of despair, positive emotions can be experienced. Strive to foster and amplify positive emotions even if you are swimming in a sea of negativity.

- Notice and savor positive events; appreciate even small ordinary occurrences, such as a good cup of coffee, a bird singing, a beautiful sunset or the scent of a flower. Amplify the good feelings by spending time reliving the event and sharing the experience with others.

- Throughout the day, appreciate something that has happened which helped you through the day; maybe a kind word or deed from someone. Don't dwell on something negative by going over it again and again; that only keeps you stuck.

- Look for the positive or what you can learn from a difficult situation. Reappraise a difficult situation: "See the silver lining", "believe something good can come of this", or, "see how things could be worse". Start with small issues, not life changing problems. For example: You have to park far away from the store door. Instead of grumbling about how far you must walk, think of it as a few minutes of more exercise to offset cravings.

- Develop an attitude of thankfulness or gratitude. Every night write down five things for which you are thankful or something you appreciate about your life. There is always something to appreciate: Do you have a roof over your head? Enough food to eat? Clothes to wear? Someone to love? Do your eyes see, your ears hear, your tongue taste, are you able to walk? Be thankful for what you do have, there are always others in the world who don't have the physical capabilities or material belongings that you do.

- Reflect on your personal strengths and resources. Remind yourself of your worth and your good qualities: dependability, being a good friend, kindness, compassion, courage, humanity, generosity, capacity to love, loyalty, leadership, faith, enthusiasm.

- Practice acts of kindness and forgiveness, using forbearance, patience, compassion and tolerance towards others. Forgiveness can be hard when you have been wronged, but it is something you do for yourself, not the other person. Get outside of yourself by volunteering to help others.

> *"Forgiveness is giving up hope*
> *that the past could have been any different."*
> Oprah Winfrey

Activity: Use the A-B-C-D Method to reframe your thoughts and beliefs.

This method is used by Cognitive Behavioral Therapists to assist their patients in changing stress producing thought patterns called Cognitive Distortions. The goal is to change your underlying beliefs about events:

Activating Event: What happened? What was the initial trigger? State the "facts" of what happened without any interpretation of the event, just who, what, where, and when.

Belief: What are you telling yourself about this event? How are you interpreting what happened? What is your perception of the situation?

Consequence: What is your emotional consequence or negative feeling resulting from your perception or interpretation of the event and your underlying belief? Often these negative feelings will trigger a craving to smoke.

Dispute: Is there an error in your thinking? Is there something from your past that in influencing how you see the situation now? Could there be another way of looking at this event instead of how you are viewing it?

Challenge any self-statement that is irrational or unrealistic such as:

- Jumping to conclusions about the behavior of another person without knowing the reason behind their actions. Don't take things personally without supporting evidence; you are not a mind reader; often the actions of another have nothing to do with you. *"My friend is ignoring me because I'm quitting."*

- Exaggeration of frequency or severity of stressors (catastrophizing): "This is *the WORST situation ever, I'll NEVER be able to handle it."*

- Black and white thinking or categorizing experiences into one of two extremes such as being 100 percent right or 100 percent wrong: *"I'm a failure because I smoked one cigarette, I'll NEVER be able to quit."*

- Imperative: *"I SHOULDN'T be such a failure."* or *"I SHOULD do better."* This keeps you stuck in a guilt cycle. Let go of expectations. Allow yourself to make mistakes.

Examples: You go to a party where others are smoking and you are offered a cigarette (activating event). Your belief or thought is, *"This is when I enjoy smoking the most but I quit smoking and I shouldn't want to smoke but I really want one. I can't have fun without smoking."* Your emotional consequence is a feeling of depravation of not being able to smoke, guilt about wanting to smoke or social pressure to fit in. With thoughts like this, it is easy to say *"yes"*.

Dispute your thoughts: *"Yes, I used to enjoy smoking at parties, however, I'm not deprived, and I can enjoy myself without smoking. I have nothing to feel guilty about and no one cares if I smoke or not. I can chose to say 'no' and have a good time smoke-free."*

Another example: You have asked your spouse to help you with a chore and s/he says *"no"* and a fight ensues (activating event). Your belief is, *"S/he SHOULDN'T treat me this way, s/he ALWAYS picks a fight with me to avoid helping me with chores."* The emotional consequence is anger which triggers a craving to smoke.

Dispute your thoughts: *"I love my spouse and s/he often is helpful. Maybe there is something else going on that has nothing to do with me as the reason why s/he doesn't want to help me right now."*

There are many other Cognitive Distortions: blame, overgeneralization, negative mental filter, discounting the positive, control error — seeing yourself as helpless and externally controlled or the opposite by feeling responsible for everything. Consult a professional therapist for additional help.

Avoid Weight Gain. Smokers who are overly concerned about gaining weight will either not try to quit or they will incorporate tools to limit weight gain into their Action Plan. Those who are not prepared, often are disturbed as the pounds add up and go back to smoking with the promise of losing the weight before quitting again. But they don't drop the weight, and now they are heavier and smoking.

Average weight gain is said to be about 10 to 12 pounds but you need to gain 50 to 100 pounds to do as much damage to your body as one pack of cigarettes. Decide it is more important for your health to stop smoking and if you can do that, you can do anything. If you do gain weight, you can lose it later on by applying some of the same tools used to "Become Smoke-Free".

Activity: What will you do to limit any weight gain?

There are eight reasons why you might gain weight. Which apply to you and which strategies will you try?

1. A change in metabolism can account for three to six pounds. About 70 percent of weight gain is due to an increase in calorie consumption, not metabolism.

- Exercise, walk twenty minutes more per day than you normally do.

2. Smoking can inhibit hunger. This may be because smokers hold food in their stomachs longer than non-smokers, or it may be that nicotine affects the appetite/satiety hormones. After quitting you may feel hungrier than before.

- Have small, low-calorie, high fiber snacks throughout the day. Include some protein and drink water.

- Nicotine Replacement Products and/or Bupropion can act as an appetite suppressant and limit weight gain.

3. Withdrawing from nicotine can cause changes in your blood sugar which can cause you to crave sugar.

- Substitute raw fruit and vegetables for pastries, candy bars and junk food.

4. You may eat more food as a substitution for the hand-to-mouth motion of smoking or as an oral fixation.

- Stock up on low-fat crunchy foods, keep healthy snacks available. Increase your intake of vegetables.

- Cut a straw the size of a cigarette or use a pretzel stick and "pretend" to smoke it. Sip water frequently. Use the nicotine inhaler.

5. Using food as a reward for not smoking.

- Find other rewards than food. Stay conscious about the amount of food you are eating. See page 21 for ideas of different rewards.

6. Eating more to delay having the "after a meal" craving. A cigarette at the end of a meal is like a period at the end of a sentence – it tells you when to stop.

- Only eat when hungry. Stop eating once you are full. Leave the table immediately. Go brush your teeth, have a breath mint, chew gum. Use a smaller plate.

- Immediately clear the table and hand wash the dishes. It is hard to smoke with wet hands.

- Keep a Food Diary. Before you eat, write down what you are going to eat, where you are, what you are doing and how you are feeling; similar to your Tobacco Use Record (see page 32).

7. Food tastes and smells better once you have quit.

- Eat slower, put your fork down in between bites. Savor the flavor of each bite. Decide how much you will eat before you start and don't take seconds.

8. Emotional eating: Using food as a substitute for not dealing with feelings and emotional needs. To escape from boredom, tension, depression, stress. Your most vulnerable times are with: Hunger, Anger (Alcohol, and Anxiety), Loneliness, and Tired: HALT and take care of your emotional needs.

- Continue your Food Diary, paying particular attention to how you are feeling when you are eating. Only eat when you are hungry. Learn the difference between hunger and emotional eating. When the desire to eat comes up, have an apple or some other healthy food. If you are having true hunger, you will eat the apple. If you don't want the apple, what need, other than hunger, do you need to address?

Develop an ICE Plan (In Case of Emergency)

The easiest way to never relapse is to never be around cigarettes. To relapse, cigarettes have to be available. Treat them as the poison they are, and avoid contact as much as possible. This is hard to do since cigarettes are as close as the nearest store or gas station, so have a plan in place to handle emergencies or when a craving seems to come from "out of the blue".

By now your common smoking habits are gone and yet seemingly out of nowhere, you get an intense craving. An "out of the blue" craving is a memory your brain has picked up on. The trigger is related to something in your environment, to an emotion, and/or represents a time or activity when you used to smoke.

Avoiding all triggers is unrealistic since some situations or emotions may be so infrequent it would be hard to foresee all possibilities but your brain remembers the connection with smoking even if you consciously don't. You are most likely to relapse in situations for which you are not prepared. Your Tobacco Use Record only covered a short period of time. Sometimes you cannot consciously identify the reason or the environmental trigger for the craving; all you know is that you just want to smoke. But there can be clues that you are walking in a field of landmines if you stay alert and diligent.

Identify early warning signs.

Have you ever ended a bad relationship but after a few months you are lonely and miss him/her? You think about the happy times together, and his/her good qualities. Before you know it, you call to get together but at this reunion you remember the reasons why the two of you are not a match and say, *"What was I thinking?"* and walk away.

The same thing happens with your cigarettes. You start thinking of how much you enjoyed smoking, and forget their negative traits and how hard it was to quit. You start romancing the idea of having "just one" again, maybe as a treat. But it isn't so easy to walk away after a reunion with nicotine.

Watch what you are saying to yourself. When the thought of a cigarette comes up, are you romancing the idea of being able to have one? What thoughts, or feelings might lead you back to smoking? Examples of these are:

"Oh, this is when I really enjoyed smoking."

"I miss the smell of my cigarettes, blow the smoke my way."

"I can control smoking."

"Nobody's going to know."

"I don't have any other way to relieve my stress."

"I can't have a good time without smoking."

"It's my only vice left."

"One won't hurt" is a common warning sign. Don't believe it. You are not more powerful than nicotine and you can't control a physical addiction. Remind yourself what a powerful hold nicotine has had on your survival instinct.

Besides, one cigarette will "hurt" you. Review the physical effects of just one cigarette: Your blood pressure increases. Your heart rate increases. Your bronchial tubes constrict making your lungs work harder. The amount of carbon monoxide in your system doubles and prevents oxygen from reaching your vital organs. The temperature of your hands and feet decrease.

How can you reframe these types of thoughts or what can you say instead? Think about quitting in a different way:

"One cigarette is too many and 1000 are not enough."

"I'm a puff away from a pack a day."

"NOPE: Not One Puff Ever."

"Let a slip slide."

Focus on your long-term positive "Benefits of Being Smoke-Free" instead of the temporary short-term pleasure of smoking "just one".

Identify high risk situations. As mentioned in Step One, (see page 36) nicotine affects the part of your brain that scans, analyzes and interprets your environment. After quitting, the first time you . . . (*name an activity where you normally smoked*) without having a cigarette, an intense craving could be triggered. Plan ahead for those "first times": The first time in a bar, going over to a smoking buddy's house, being in an airport, on your annual vacation or family reunion.

Do you live in a State that still allows smoking in restaurants and bars where the combination of alcohol, being around other smokers and having a good time can lead to a relapse?

If you live in a State that has banned public smoking, how will you handle it when traveling to another State where smoking is allowed? Or your annual vacation or business convention, that has, in the past, always included your cigarettes?

Social situations are often a place where temptation lurks:

- If you can't avoid an event, bring along a support person. Avoid alcohol. If someone lights up, excuse yourself and go to the bathroom, go say *"hello"* to someone else—anything to get around sitting there while someone is smoking.

- If you're at a social event and feel tempted, leave if you are able to do so and protect yourself from caving in to saying, *"I'm just going to have one."* You could always develop an upset stomach for which you need to leave to take care of.

- Do you still go out to the "butt hut" or the smoking area on your work breaks with your smoking buddies? Some smokers might try to sabotage your success and won't take *"no"* for an answer. Give your reason(s), change the subject, or try some humor to deflect their temptations.

What situations happen in your life, that aren't listed, which could cause you to be tempted to smoke?

Activity: Create your ICE Plan.

What are some of your early warning signs and high risk situations? If you have quit and then relapsed, what caused you to pick up that first cigarette? Where did you get the cigarette? Did you buy a pack, bum one or did someone give it to you? What did you say to yourself to make it OK to smoke it? Use your answers to find new solutions to avoid relapsing this time.

Write down the answers to the following questions in your notebook, so you can read back your ICE plan when you need to. Have it all written out so you don't have to think about what to do when that "out of the blue" craving hits you.

- What can you say to yourself to talk yourself out of caving in?

- How can you change your behavior to avoid smoking? What can you do instead? Where is a safe place for you to be where smoking isn't allowed?

- Who can you call for help? Call someone who is understanding and will not judge you when you are being tempted to smoke. See page 82 for a list of your supporters. Are there some saboteurs you need to avoid for a while?

- What tools in your Action Plan helped in similar situations or that you used in previous attempts?

- What life skills do you need to work on? (i.e. stress, anger or time management, weight control, alcohol and/or substance dependence)

If You Have Finished This Book and Are Smoke-Free. Congratulations on "Becoming Smoke-Free"! I knew you could do it. "Becoming Smoke-Free" may be one of the hardest things you have ever done. Be proud of yourself for all the effort you put forth. Congratulations again!

If you quit but have relapsed. Congratulate yourself for completing a "practice run". Don't view this "practice run" as a failure but a learning experience. By reframing this attempt as a "practice run", you will discover where the weakness is in your Plan. Besides you did have a success – look at how many cigarettes you didn't smoke and how much money you saved. (20 cigarettes per day is 140 cigarettes per week or 1400 puffs avoided!)

Look at everything you tried that did work. Look at all the tools you did develop which did help. Don't reinvent the wheel but refine it. Decide if you need to add more tools to your quitting toolbox or if you need to replace what didn't work. Finding out a particular method doesn't work for you helps to lead you to what will. Evaluate the different areas to see where your strengths lie and where you need to improve on your Action Plan: social, physical, emotional, environment and/or thought patterns.

Look at the circumstances that led to that first cigarette. What happened? Where did you get the cigarette? What rationalization did you use to give yourself permission to smoke? Did you follow your ICE plan? If not, why not? Are you willing to write your "pre-commitment" check or did you not make that pre-commitment? (See page 73).

Decide whether you are ready to set a new Quit Date now or if you will try again later.

Start this book all over again. What didn't you do that could have helped? What advice did you ignore? Appendix H (see page 162) is a list of Activities in this book. Which ones did you not do? Resolve to do them for your next effort.

Talk to a Tobacco Treatment Specialist to revise your Action Plan. As specialists in behavior modification, a professional can help you to uncover what is missing in your quitting puzzle. Call 1-800- QUIT-NOW for your local state quit line.

Finally, reassess your desire to quit. Be honest with yourself. Do you really want to "Become Smoke-Free" or were you doing it for someone else or because of outside pressures? There is no right or wrong answer; the purpose is to find out where you need help. Often it is only by looking back and examining the situation that you see what you couldn't before. Hindsight is always 20/20 vision.

Learn what does not work:

- Relying on willpower alone. Nicotine has hijacked the survival instinct part of your brain which is stronger than the thinking part of the brain (willpower).
- Mentally beating yourself up or scolding yourself. Let go of both shame and/or guilt. It's not your fault. Becoming Smoke-Free is HARD work.
- Thinking there is something wrong with you. It's not uncommon for a smoker to quit many times before being successful. The blame belongs to how cigarettes have been manipulated to be as addictive as possible.
- Not trying one more time.

"Never, never, never give up."
Winston Churchill

If you haven't quit. Did you read through this book without doing any of the activities or spend any time writing down the answers to the questions asked? This is fine if you plan to start over again and take action this time.

Don't say you *"tried and it didn't work"* if you are unwilling to take time with each Step, to get a notebook, write down the answers to the questions asked and do the activities. Just as you cannot learn to play the piano by reading a book, you will not change your behavior unless you take action and practice.

Commit to start at Step One and do the activities. You will be glad you did, because you will find that quitting is much easier than you think when you are prepared. Take as much time as you need with each Step, only moving on when you are ready. I know you will be successful and you will be proud of yourself for the rest of your life.

Challenge for Step Four:

You have stopped smoking; the challenge now is to remain smoke-free.

Honor your journey and how far you have come. Rejoice in regaining your freedom. Feel empowered by accomplishing something so difficult and celebrate each smoke-free day.

Appendices

Assess Your Nicotine Dependence*

Add up your score from the following questions:

How soon after you wake up do you smoke your first cigarette?

- After 60 minutes: 0 pt.
- 31-60 minutes: 1 pt.
- 6-30 minutes: 2 pts.
- Within 5 minutes: 3 pts.

Do you find it difficult to refrain from smoking in places where it is forbidden?

- No: 0 pt.
- Yes: 1 pt.

Which cigarette would you hate most to give up?

- The first in the morning: 1 pt.
- Any other: 0 pt.

How many cigarettes per day do you smoke?

- 10 cigarettes or less: 0 pt.
- 11-20 cigarettes: 1 pt.
- 21-30 cigarettes: 2 pts.
- 31 or more cigarettes: 3 pts.

Do you smoke more frequently during the first hours after awakening than during the rest of the day?

- No: 0 pt.
- Yes: 1 pt.

Do you smoke even if you are so ill that you are in bed most of the day?

- No: 0 pt.

- Yes: 1 pt.

Total Score _____

Your level of dependence on nicotine is:

0-2 Very low dependence

3-4 Low dependence

5 Medium dependence

6-7 High dependence

8-10 Very high dependence

Scores under 5: Your level of nicotine dependence is still low. You should act now before your level of dependence increases. Even with a low score, you may be physically addicted to nicotine.

Score of 5-6: Your level of nicotine dependence is moderate. If you don't quit soon, your level of dependence on nicotine will increase until you may be seriously addicted. Act now to end your dependence on nicotine.

Score over 7: Your level of dependence is high. You are not in control of your smoking — it is in control of you! When you make the decision to quit, you may want to talk with your doctor about nicotine replacement therapy or other medications to help you break your addiction.

*Fagerstrom Test for Nicotine Dependence

List of Resources

Free Services:

1-800-Quit-Now: National Telephone Quit Line

The Tobacco Control Research Branch of the National Cancer Institute: www.smokefree.gov

The author's blog:
http://stopsmokingstayquit.blogspot.com/

The American Legacy Foundation:
http://www.becomeanex.org/

American Cancer Society:
http://www.cancer.org/Healthy/StayAwayfromTobacco/
GuidetoQuittingSmoking/index?from=fast

For smokeless tobacco users:
http://www.chewfree.com/
or http://www.killthecan.org/

Nicotine Anonymous:
http://www.nicotine-anonymous.org/

Resources for military personnel and family:
http://www.ucanquit2.org/

American Heart Association:
http://www.heart.org/HEARTORG/GettingHealthy/Quit
Smoking/QuitSmoking_UCM_001085_SubHomePage.jsp.

Tobacco Dependence Program from the University of Medicine and Dentistry of New Jersey:
http://www.tobaccoprogram.org/quitguides.htm

National Institute of Drug Abuse:
http://www.nida.nih.gov/ResearchReports/Nicotine/Nico
tine.html

Advocacy:

Tobacco-Free Kids: http://www.tobaccofreekids.org/

Action on Smoking and Health: http://www.ash.org/

Americans for Non-Smokers Rights:
http://www.no-smoke.org/

UCSF Center for Tobacco Control Research and
Education: http://www.smokefreemovies.ucsf.edu/

College Campus Campaign:
http://www.tobaccofreeu.org/

Various Chemicals in Tobacco Smoke

There are about 600 chemicals in a cigarette which when burned create over 7,000 chemicals in the smoke; many are cancer causing, cancer promoting, poisonous or irritants. Every cigarette smoked may cause one genetic mutation leading to cancer. Twenty cigarettes per day would equal 146,000 gene mutations over 20 years which is why smoking is a leading cause of 30% of all cancers. Many have fallen victim to a marketing campaign promoting "organic" or "natural" tobacco cigarettes. They are just as deadly and actually contain a higher amount of nicotine.

Acetone: Used as nail polish remover.

Acetylene: Used with oxygen in welding torches.

Aluminum: Metal.

Ammonia compounds are used in household cleaners and fertilizers. They are added to increase the pH level of nicotine to increase the speed it hits your brain. Fast absorption increases its addictive nature.

Aromatic Amines: 4-Aminobiphenyl, 2-Naphthylamine. Cause cancer.

Arsenic: A metallic substance, poisonous to all life. The human body can build up a tolerance to arsenic.

Benzene: A cancer causing poison that interferes with cellular metabolism. Used in Napalm and gasoline.

Bronchodilators: Added to expand the airways in the lungs making it easier for smoke to pass into your lungs.

Butane: Cigarette lighter fuel.

Cadmium: A cancer causing metal used in car batteries. It accumulates in the lungs, damages the liver, kidneys and brain, and has an adverse effect on the protective immune system. It can stay in the body for 10 years.

Carbon Monoxide: Same gas that comes from the tailpipe of your car. It deprives the red blood cells of oxygen by binding to the cells in your blood system 230 times faster than oxygen where it can remain for up to six hours. Related to heart attacks and strokes. Affects non-smokers in side-stream smoke coming off the tip of a cigarette.

Chromium: Used to make steel.

DDT: Insecticide banned by most industrialized nations.

Ethanol: Alcohol.

Flavorings: Used to mask the harshness of tobacco; includes menthol which cools and numbs your throat to reduce irritation and make the smoke feel smoother. Children are attracted to different flavors. Banned by the FDA in cigarettes, the Tobacco companies switched to making flavored cigarillos and electronic cigarettes.

Formaldehyde: Used to embalm dead bodies. Damages lungs, skin and digestive tract. Causes cancer.

Hexamine: Used in barbecue lighter fluid.

Hydrazine: Used in jet and rocket fuel.

Hydrogen Cyanide: Poison used in the gas chamber and chemical weapons. EPA standards of 10 parts per million are generally safe. Cigarette smoke produces an average 1600 parts per million.

Lead: Found in old paint and leaded gasoline. Stunts growth. Damages brain, kidneys and nervous system.

Mercury: Heavy metal found in thermometers which affects the central nervous system.

Methane: Sewer or swamp gas.

Methanol: Rocket fuel.

Methoprene: Insecticide used to kill fleas on animals.

Naphthalene: Mothball chemical.

Nickel: Heavy metal affecting central nervous system.

Nicotine: A poisonous alkaloid that is the main active ingredient of tobacco. Originally used as an insecticide but outlawed as too toxic. Levels have been manipulated by the Tobacco Companies to make it as physically addictive as possible.

Nitro-benzene: Gasoline additive.

Nitrous Oxide Phenols: Used as a disinfectant.

Phenol: Toilet bowl disinfectant. Causes irritation of the skin, eyes and mucous membranes.

Polonium-210: Cancer causing radioactive substance. Used in nuclear weapons. The source is the fertilizer used on tobacco leaves. Smoking 30 cigarettes a day for a year is the equivalent to 300 chest x-rays.

Polycyclic Aromatic Hydrocarbons (PAH): Includes Benzanthracene and Benezopyrene which is one of the most potent cancer-causing chemicals known.

Propylene Glycol: Helps deliver nicotine to the brain.

Stearic Acid: Candle wax.

Sugar: Added to make tobacco easier to inhale. It forms acetaldehyde which enhances the addictive nature of nicotine.

Tar: A particulate matter used for paving streets. Has dozens of compounds. Some are toxic, some are cancer-causing. Tar cools inside the lungs, forming a sticky mass that damages delicate lung tissue. The average pack-a-day smoker inhales a cup of tar into their lungs every year.

Tobacco-Specific Nitrosamines (TSNA): Cancer causing chemicals created by curing and heating process, humidity and type of fertilizer used. American cigarettes are made from blended tobaccos which are flue-cured and have higher levels of these cancer-causing substances.

Toluene: Found in paint thinner, embalmers glue and used as an industrial solvent. Depresses the central nervous system.

Turpentine: Toxic chemical used in paint stripper.

Ventilated filters are the holes in the filter which cause a smoker to inhale more robustly, drawing cancer-causing substances deeper into the lungs.

Vinyl Chloride: Cancer causing substance found in PVC pipes and tennis shoes.

Summary of Cessation Medications

The US Public Health Service's 2008 Clinical Practice Guideline, "Treating Tobacco Use and Dependence", recommends that every individual attempting to quit be offered cessation medications.

However, every medication, whether it is over-the-counter or a prescription medication, has both risks and benefits, and possible side effects. It is important you discuss these risks and benefits with your doctor, along with your medical and mental health history, other substance use and current medications, previous quit attempts and the amount you smoke. These factors will determine the right medication or combination of medications which are appropriate for you.

There are seven FDA approved first line medications for smoking cessation. They fall into two categories: medications containing nicotine (NRT-nicotine gum, lozenge, patch, inhaler and nasal spray) and non-nicotine medications (Bupropion and Chantix™). Often a combination of medications works better than a single one. Combinations usually consist of one long-acting medication combined with a short-acting medication such as:

- The Patch with either the gum, lozenge, nasal spray or inhaler.

- Bupropion with either the gum, lozenge, nasal spray or inhaler.

Less common combinations are:

- Bupropion with the Patch and a short acting NRT-Gum, Lozenge, Nasal Spray or Inhaler.

- Bupropion and Chantix™.

- Chantix™ with a short-acting NRT-Gum, Lozenge, Nasal Spray or Inhaler.

Not all dosing recommendations listed are FDA approved and are not contained in the current product labeling information. The most effective dose varies by individual. Medication recommendations change as new research is published, please schedule an appointment with your doctor or nurse to discuss the proper use of cessation medications.

Nicotine Replacement Therapy (NRT) stabilizes your brain by occupying the nicotinic acetylcholine receptors, the same receptors that nicotine from smoking occupies (see page 34). No NRT provides the same level of nicotine you get from freebasing nicotine by smoking, so it is important to use enough NRT to reduce your withdrawal symptoms and curb your cravings. The nicotine inhaler and spray are only available by prescription and will give the highest doses of nicotine but still far short of smoking.

Short-acting NRT (gum, lozenge, inhaler and nasal spray) can be used while you are still smoking and can be used in place of smoking a cigarette. This will decrease the number of cigarettes you smoke in anticipation of your actual Quit Date.

Since every smoker is different in the strength of their nicotine addiction, instead of following an arbitrary reduction schedule, I suggest staying with a NRT dosage until you have been able to go two full weeks without a major craving or slip before even considering tapering down a level.

"Dose them to the level of their addiction."
Dr. Richard Hurt, The Mayo Clinic

All Nicotine Replacement Products should be disposed in a safe manner to avoid accidental poisoning of pets and young children.

The Nicotine Patch is similar to a Band-Aid and delivers nicotine through your skin for a steady source of nicotine. It is easy to use and is applied just once a day. Patches may be placed anywhere on the upper body, including arms and back, rotating the Patch site each time a new one is applied. It can take two to six hours to reach the full strength. It is available over-the-counter and as a generic medication.

There are few side effects. Some people are allergic to the adhesive used to hold the Patch onto the skin. Switching to a different manufacturer may solve this issue. If the skin irritation is minor, a hydrocortisone cream can be used. Some people will experience vivid dreams and/or insomnia. You can use the 16 hour Patch and place it on in the morning to reduce these effects.

Dosage for the Patch: The Patch comes in various strengths, from 25 mg down to 7 mg and can be left on for 16 to 24 hours. The initial dosage for the Patch will depend upon how much you smoke and can be adjusted accordingly:

- If you smoke less than 10 cigarettes per day, start with a 14 mg Patch.

- If you smoke more than 10 cigarettes per day, use a 21 to 25 mg Patch.

- If you smoke 21 to 39 cigarettes per day, use two Patches together equal to 28 to 35 mg. (Two 14 mg Patches equals 28 mg or a 21 mg plus 14 mg equals 35 mg).

- If you smoke more than 40 cigarettes a day, use two 21 mg Patches or a dose of 42 mg a day.

It is designed to wean you off nicotine by lowering the dosage every two weeks. After your Quit Date, taper your dosage every two to four weeks in increments of 7 to 14 mg based on your level of urges, withdrawal symptoms and comfort level.

Nicotine Gum is a sugar-free gum-like substance that contains nicotine and is absorbed through the lining of your mouth. It is not to be constantly chewed like regular gum but chewed just long enough until a peppery or tingling sensation appears and then it is parked between your cheek and gums. When the tingling sensation fades, chew it again to reactivate the tingling sensation and rotate it to a different part of your mouth.

The Gum is convenient to use and can be used on an as needed basis. It works faster than the Patch and satisfies the oral craving. It can be effective with smokeless tobacco users. Don't eat or drink 15 minutes before using or during its use because it will interfere with the adsorption of the nicotine.

It is available over-the-counter and as a generic in a variety of flavors: cherry, orange, mint and regular. Some people find any flavor has the unpleasant taste of nicotine.

Side effects include jaw pain. Avoid using the gum if you have dental problems or TMJ syndrome. Nausea can occur if you swallow the nicotine released by the Gum.

Dosage for Nicotine Gum: It comes in two strengths, 4 mg and 2 mg.

- If you smoke more than 20 cigarettes a day and smoke within 30 minutes of waking: use 4 mg Gum.

- If you smoke less than 20 cigarettes a day and smoke at least 30 minutes after waking: use 2 mg Gum.

You need to use it frequently during the day to obtain adequate nicotine levels if used alone or it can be used on an as needed basis if used in combination with the Patch. Use one to two pieces of Gum every one to two hours (about 10 to 12 pieces a day). Taper off as tolerated.

Nicotine Lozenge and Mini Lozenge deliver nicotine through the lining of the mouth as it dissolves. The efficacy and side effects are related to the amount used.

The Lozenge is available over-the-counter, is easy to use, convenient and can be used on an as needed basis. It delivers 25 percent more nicotine than the Gum. It may help with weight control as an appetite suppressant.

The Lozenge is placed between your cheek and gum. It can be very slow to dissolve, up to one and a half hours. The

Mini-lozenge works quicker, taking 45 minutes to dissolve. Don't eat or drink 15 minutes before or during use because it interferes with the adsorption. Don't chew or swallow the Lozenge. Side effects include nausea, hiccups and heartburn.

Dosage for Lozenge and Mini-lozenge: Available in 2 and 4 mg, same as the gum.

- If you smoke more than 20 cigarettes a day and smoke within 30 minutes of waking: use 4 mg Lozenge.

- If you smoke less than 20 cigarettes a day and smoke at least 30 minutes after waking: use 2 mg Lozenge.

Use one to two Lozenges every one to two hours (about 10 to 12 pieces a day). If used in combination with the Patch, use the Lozenge on an "as needed" basis for breakthrough cravings. Taper off as tolerated.

Nicotine Nasal Spray delivers nicotine through the lining of the nose when sprayed into each nostril. Unlike nasal sprays used to relieve allergy symptoms, the Nicotine Nasal Spray is not meant to be sniffed. It is to be sprayed against the lining or side of each nostril once or twice an hour, not to exceed five times an hour.

The Nasal Spray has the fastest delivery of medicinal nicotine of the currently available NRT products. Its use allows flexible dosing and can be used in response to stress or strong urges to smoke. The Spray requires a prescription because of the possibility of nicotine dependency.

Nose and eye irritation is common. These usually disappear within one week. It can be sprayed under the tongue or between the cheek and gums, but has an unpleasant taste.

Dosage for Nicotine Nasal Spray: One spray in each nostril one to two times/hour (up to five times per hour or 40 times per day). An average user will use 14-15 doses per day. Taper as tolerated.

Nicotine Inhaler is a plastic cylinder containing a nicotine cartridge that you puff on. You don't need to inhale deeply to achieve an effect. The nicotine is absorbed through the mucosa in your mouth and not through the lungs. Puffing must be done frequently, far more often than with a cigarette. Each cartridge is designed for 80 puffs over 20 minutes of use.

The Nicotine Inhaler mimics the hand-to-mouth behavior of smoking and has few side effects. It can cause mouth or throat irritation.

A prescription is required.

Dosage for Nicotine Inhaler: Minimum of six cartridges per day, up to a maximum of 16 cartridges per day unless used in combination therapy with the Patch, then use on an "as needed" basis. Taper off use as tolerated.

Combination Nicotine Replacement Therapy (NRT) is effective for highly addicted smokers where the use of the Nicotine Patch is matched to the level of the smoker's addiction. It is used in combination with short acting nicotine (Gum, Lozenge, Inhaler or Spray) on an "as needed" basis for those times when the cravings are particularly strong. If the individual has used either NRT or Bupropion alone and has not been successful, a combination of NRT and Bupropion can be recommended.

The advantages of using Combination NRT is that it gives you a continuous level of nicotine in your body along with being able to use another product on an "as needed" basis to give you more nicotine when you really need it by using two different delivery systems. It is more effective than using only one medication.

The downside is that it is more expensive than using one NRT and it may increase the risk of getting too much nicotine. If you start to feel nauseated, get a headache, or "buzzed", take off the Patch and don't use any more nicotine until the effects wear off.

Dosage for Combination NRT:

- Dose the Patch as described above.

- Then use one of the following: 2 mg Gum, 2 mg Lozenge, Inhaler or Nasal Spray on an "as needed" basis. The doses are all adjustable depending on the level of urges and withdrawal symptoms. Adjust the Patch dosage to a higher dosage if you are using too much of the other medicinal nicotine product.

Bupropion (Zyban ™) is a medication that does not contain nicotine. It was originally developed as an anti-depressant. Researchers noticed that some people quit smoking when using it as an anti-depressant. It works on the reward center or pleasure pathway in the brain and reduces the craving to smoke.

It is available by prescription only in an easy to use pill form. It can be started while you are still smoking. It can be used in Combination Therapy with Nicotine Replacement Products or Chantix™, and may help in preventing weight gain.

It should not be used if you have certain medical conditions or take certain medications. There is a slight risk of seizure (1:1000) which is increased if you have a history of seizures, significant head trauma, brain injury, or if you suffer from anorexia or bulimia.

Bupropion has a FDA boxed warning. Read product information for safety issues and possible side effects including anxiety, rash, insomnia, headache or dry mouth.

Dosage for Bupropion:

- Start medication one week prior to Quit Date.

- Take doses at least eight hours apart. 150 mg once daily for three days, then 150 mg twice daily for four days, then stop smoking.

- Continue at 150 mg twice a day for 12 weeks, or longer if necessary as prescribed by your doctor.

No need to taper off and it can be stopped abruptly.

Chantix™ (Varenicline) is a non-nicotine medication that has a dual action. It partially blocks nicotine from attaching to the nicotinic acetylcholine receptors in your brain and also allows the receptor to release some dopamine. It reduces the enjoyment received from smoking. It can be started while you are still smoking.

It is available by prescription only in an easy to use pill form. There are no known drug interactions, however you should decrease the amount of alcohol you drink.

Nausea is common. Taking it with food will help. Some people experience vivid dreams. The evening dose should be taken several hours before bedtime to relieve the dreams. If your kidney function is impaired then the dose must be adjusted.

Chantix™ has a FDA boxed warning; read product information for safety issues and possible side effects such as nausea, vivid or unusual dreams, constipation or gas.

Dosage for Chantix™:

- Start medication one week prior to Quit Date. Take 0.5 mg once daily for three days, then 0.5 mg twice daily for four days then stop smoking.

- On your Quit Date take 1.0 mg twice daily for 11 weeks. One dose of 1.0 mg may be used for less heavily addicted smokers and/or users who want to lessen the side effects.

- If you are not smoking at the end of 12 weeks, you may continue taking 1.0 mg twice daily for an additional 12 weeks.

While it is not recommended by the manufacturer, if the smoker is still smoking at the end of 12 weeks, NRT can be added as a combination therapy. It can also be used in combination with Bupropion.

Second Line Medications: These are used if nothing else works.

Nortriptyline: A tricyclic anti-depressant that requires monitoring by an experienced medical prescriber because of significant side effects: dry mouth, sedation, constipation, low blood pressure, urinary symptoms.

Clonidine: A hypertensive with significant side effects: low blood pressure, dry mouth, constipation. Dosage must be tapered down when discontinuing.

Mecamylamine: Lowers blood pressure. Has considerable side effects: drowsiness, constipation and hypotension. May work by blocking the nicotinic receptors and may enhance the effect of nicotine replacement products. May be effective in combination with nicotine patch.

Websites for Cessation Medications: Some manufacturers have programs for those in financial need. Also check with your state quit line (I-800-QUIT-NOW) to see if any free or reduced cost products are available in your area.

Pfizer Pharmaceuticals, Chantix™:
http://www.chantix.com

Pfizer Pharmaceuticals, nicotine inhaler:
http://www.nicotrol.com

Novartis, nicotine gum: http://www.habitrol.com

GlaxoSmithKline, nicotine patch:
http://www.nicodermcq.com

GlaxoSmithKline, nicotine gum:
http://www.nicorette.com

Sponsored by GlaxoSmithKline:
http://www.way2quit.com/

Unproven and/or Ineffective
Products and Services

Every method will work for some individuals but no method will work for everyone. Most "stop smoking" products are worthless except for the power given them because of the placebo effect which is the belief or positive expectation it will work.

Some methods have many anecdotal stories of success, yet have no clinical trials acceptable to the Public Health Service.

Avoid any product or service that guarantees a 100 percent quit rate. It's a 100 percent guarantee they just want your money because when it comes to quitting, there is no one-size-fits-all or even one-size-fits-most!

Some products are actually dangerous and claim to be FDA approved. Check with your doctor.

Acupuncture: Anecdotal stories as to efficacy but no evidence to support efficacy as a cessation method in research studies.

E-cigarettes: A battery operated device, which vaporizes nicotine, propylene glycol, water and flavorings. Cannot be advertised as a cessation device. Anecdotal stories as to efficacy but insufficient evidence to support e-cigarettes as a cessation method. No current manufacturing standards or regulation. For more information about electronic cigarettes, read "E-cigarettes, The Good, The Bad, The Ugly, A Cessation Device or Alternative Vice" by VJ Sleight.

Hypnosis: Anecdotal stories as to efficacy but insufficient evidence to support hypnosis as a cessation method.

Lobedia: Also known as Indian tobacco, a substance chemically similar to nicotine that is used in tablets, gum and vitamins pills. Marketed as a substance to help with nicotine withdrawal. Controlled studies have not shown it to be effective. Banned by the FDA in 1993 as a cessation medication.

NicBloc: A corn syrup solution applied to the filter of a cigarette. The claim is that the solution blocks the tar and other components but no studies have shown this to be true. No effectiveness for cessation was seen over a placebo.

Silver Acetate: A crystalline substance, often an ingredient in chewing gum that is claimed to produce a repulsive taste when combined with cigarette smoke. No beneficial effects for cessation have been shown in randomized clinical studies.

Silver Nitrate: In chewing gum, mouth washes or lozenges combines with saliva in the smoker's mouth to produce a bad taste. Has not been shown to be effective.

Smokeless Tobacco or Snus: Tobacco products that are held in the mouth. Different products have varying levels of harmful components. Linked to cancers of the mouth, tongue, gums, lips and cheeks. Causes cavities, tooth loss, stained teeth and gum disease. Swallowing spit can cause heartburn, ulcers and cancers of the voice box, esophagus and parts of the throat and stomach. Increases blood pressure and heart rate. May contain more nicotine than cigarettes.

Welplex: An injection consisting of a combination of atropine, scopolamine and chlorpromazine (thorazine). This combination may cause a temporary mental break including hallucinations, heart palpitations, paranoia and possible coma. Not approved by the FDA for smoking cessation. Atropine is used to dilate the eyes. Scopolamine is used for motion sickness. Chlorpromazine is used for psychiatric disorders such as schizophrenia.

Partial List of Interactions Between Medications and Smoking*

Smoking can interfere with many different medications. Coordinate with your doctor since your dosages may need to be adjusted after you quit smoking. Your pharmacist is a good resource regarding any potential interactions.

Benzodiazepines: Smokers may have less sedation and drowsiness compared to non-smokers, which may be due to the stimulation that nicotine gives to the central nervous system.

Beta-blockers: Smoking makes the medication less effective. Smokers may need a higher dose.

Birth-Control Pills (Oral Contraceptives): There is an increased risk of heart attack, stroke and embolism. The risk increases with age (over 35 years old) and the amount smoked (15 or more cigarettes per day).

Caffeine: The level of caffeine in the blood system can double after stopping smoking.

Camptosar (Irinotecan): Smokers may need a higher dosage than a non-smoker because of the reduction in efficacy.

Clozaril (Clozapine): Smoking reduces blood levels by about 20 percent. A reduction in dosage may be needed after cessation to avoid toxicity.

Cognex (Tacrine): Blood levels in a smoker can be three times lower than in a non-smoker. Smokers will require a higher dosage.

Corticosteriods (inhaled): Smokers with asthma may have a lower response than non-smokers.

Haldol (Halperidol): Blood levels in smokers are 70 percent less than in non-smokers.

Heparin: The medication leaves the body faster in a smoker than in a non-smoker. Smokers may need a higher dosage.

Inderal (Propranolol): Medication leaves the smoker's body faster than in a non-smoker.

Insulin: Smokers may need a higher dose because the absorption of the insulin may be decreased due to the constrictive effect nicotine has on the blood vessels. Smoking may contribute to insulin resistance.

Mexitil (Mexiletine): The medicine leaves the body faster and by a greater amount in a smoker than in a non-smoker.

Luvox (Fluvoxamine): Smokers may require higher dosages than non-smokers.

Opioids: Higher doses may be required in smokers.

Requip (Ropinirole): Smokers may need a higher dosage.

Tambocor (Flecainide): Smokers require higher dosages than non-smokers.

Tarceva (Erlotinib): Smoking increases clearance from the body and decreases blood levels.

Treanda (Bendamustine): Smoking decreases levels of this medication and increases concentrations of its two active metabolites.

Theophylline: Maintenance doses are higher in smokers. A patient needs to be monitored if they either start or stop smoking. Both smoking and exposure to secondhand smoke can affect how fast the medication leaves the body.

Thorazine (Chlorpromazine): Smokers may need higher levels than non-smokers, may experience less sedation and have low blood pressure.

Tricyclic Antidepressants: There may be a possible interaction but the importance of clinical levels has not been established.

Xanax (Alprazolam): Smoking interferes with the absorption and can reduce blood levels by 50 percent.

Zyprexa (Olanzapine): Smokers may need a higher dosage because the medication is metabolized faster in a smoker.

*Adapted from: Smoking Cessation Leadership Center/Rx for Change.

The Seven "D's"

Drink water or fruit juice to help flush the nicotine out of your system. Squeeze lemon juice in your water. Limit juice due to the calories. Satisfy your oral fixation in other ways. Get a water bottle and sip water throughout the day to replace the hand-to-mouth motion of smoking. Drink herbal tea instead of coffee. Don't drink alcoholic beverages.

Deep breathing from your abdomen. Avoid shallow breathing. Lie on the floor with a piece of paper on your navel, trying to lift the paper by using your breath. Breathe deeply through your nose for five seconds, exhaling through your mouth for five seconds. This ten-second breathing cycle will slow down your heart rate and calm you down.

Do something else. Get your mind off the cigarette. Keep your hands busy. Engage in substitute activities. Play a musical instrument or computer games. Do a crossword puzzle. Read a book or magazine. Write letters. Start a new hobby or learn craft projects: Knit, crochet, needlepoint, garden, paint, sculpt. Reach for a pen and paper and doodle or sketch rather than a cigarette when answering the phone. Do house or yard work. Clean out the closets or the garage. Vacuum the floor. Organize your junk drawer. Change the oil. Give yourself or someone else a manicure or pedicure. Get your hands wet. Take a shower or splash cold water on your face. Wash your hair. Shampoo the dog or cat. Do the dishes. Brush your teeth. Balance your checkbook. Surf the Internet. Google yourself. Exercise. Go for a brisk walk. If you cannot walk outside, walk the interior of a shopping mall. Walk the dog. Go bowling, play tennis, ride a bike. Go for a swim. Lift weights. Climb a flight of stairs instead of using the elevator. Stretch, touch your toes, do jumping jacks. Park a block or two away from your destination and walk. Change your routine. Replace old habits with new ones, such as: Try tea instead of coffee. Take a five minute walk after a meal. Take a walk at your break instead of going to where you used to smoke. Sit in a different chair; avoid your "smoking" seat. Eat lunch in a new place not associated with past smoking behavior. Chew on a straw, cinnamon stick, toothpick, clove, sugarless gum or candy. Have carrot or celery sticks on hand. Try eating unshelled, unsalted sunflower seeds. Eat one at a time. Go someplace you can't smoke such as the library, a museum, or the movies.

Delay. Wait it out; a craving will often fade and disappear in a few minutes. Count to 300 slowly or count backwards from 300 to 1. Write down all your reasons for being smoke-free. Say to yourself, *"I'll think of cigarettes five minutes from now"*; then go do something else and soon, the thought of your cigarettes will be gone. Don't say that you won't think about smoking because then that will be all that you will think about. Talk yourself out of it, tell yourself, *"This isn't going to last, it is only temporary"*. Take a nap. Remember the craving will go away whether or not you smoke.

Discuss with a friend. Find helping relationships and support. Call or text a non-smoking support person or your quit buddy. Go to a Nicotine Anonymous meeting. Your best support may be someone who has kept you at a distance because you smoke. Seek out others who are going through the quitting process now, or have successfully quit in the past. Avoid people who will tempt you to return to smoking, or try and sabotage your success. Bet someone you won't smoke. Put money in a jar each day. Forfeit it if you smoke. Keep the money if you don't smoke. Try it for a week then extend it to a month. Tell everyone you are trying to quit and you are making a Plan. Ask for their support. Be specific about how they can help you. Join BecomeAnEx.org and get support from others on-line.

Distract your thoughts. Change the way you think about smoking and get your mind off the cigarette. Listen to what you are saying to yourself about quitting; change your self-talk. When the thought of a cigarette comes up, deliberately choose to focus your mind on something else. Kiss someone. Wake up each morning and say, *"I'm proud I made it another day smoke-free."* Remember *"NOPE: Not One Puff Ever"*. Or, *"I'm a puff away from a pack a day"*.

Repeat positive affirmations such as: *"I love the thought of being smoke-free."* Or, *"I choose to be smoke-free."* Or, *"I look better, I smell better. I'm saving a ton of money"* Remind yourself of a difficult situation where you overcame the temptation to smoke and tell yourself, *"I've done it before and I can do it again."* Ask yourself, *"Do I really want this cigarette?"* Or, *"How will this cigarette help?"* Think of a negative image of smoking. Imagine this whenever the urge comes up. For example: A burn a hole in a favorite outfit, yellow teeth, 20 terrorists (cigarettes) in a pack trying to kill you, how breathless you are after exercising or walking up a flight of stairs.

Don't smoke no matter what. Prepare for tempting situations by mentally visualizing yourself handling the situation without smoking. Remind yourself of what's really important and it's not the cigarette. Think of your pre-commitment deal you made with yourself. Imagine writing that check. Continue to carry your Reasons to Quit Card and review as often as possible. Carry a picture of a child or grandchild who you want to be alive for in the future. Or a picture of someone who has passed — vow to quit smoking in their memory. Look at the picture every time a craving comes up. Remember, thinking and dreaming about a cigarette is not the same as craving it. Be careful to identify excuses. There are no good reasons to smoke, only excuses.

List of Activities and Visual Aids

Activities:

Step One: Build Motivation

Make two lists: "Benefits of Becoming Smoke-Free" and "Consequences of Continuing to Smoke" 9

Figure out how much money you will save by not smoking 10

Make a Reasons to Quit Card 16

Reasons for Smoking 17

Figure out how many cigarette puffs smoked 29

Start a Tobacco Use Record 31

Take the Nicotine Dependency Test 38

Decide how you will handle nicotine withdrawals 43

Answer the following: *"I smoke because . . . "* 43

Uncover your underlying fears 46

Releasing fear meditation 48

Make two lists: "Benefits of Smoking" and "Consequences of Quitting" 49

Reframe each of your beliefs and fears 51

Compare and contrast lists 55

Step Two: Create Your Action Plan

Choose a Quit Date 60

Figure out how much time you spend smoking 62

Make a Smoking Corner and Smoke by the Clock....... 63

Start tracking your common triggers............................ 66

Create an Action Plan... 66

Decide on different strategies to prepare you 70

Make a list of support people with their phone
numbers and people to avoid... 82

Step Three: Your First Week Smoke-Free

Recognize the symptoms of physical withdrawal
from nicotine and develop strategies for coping.......... 88

Make a Nicotine Withdrawal and Coping Strategies
Card... 91

Five steps to train your brain to think of smoking
in a different way. 96

Step Four: Prevent Relapse

If you have relapsed before, was it a short-term or
long-term relapse and what was the reason? 104

Understand how stress may affect you. Make a list
of the symptoms that apply to you. 109

Decide how you can relieve your stress. 111

Develop tools to change your attitude....................... 116

Use the A-B-C-D Method 118

What will you do to limit any weight gain? 121

Create your ICE Plan. 127

Visual Aids:

"Benefits of Becoming Smoke-Free" and
"Consequences of Continuing to Smoke". 9

Chart of cost of smoking for day, 1 year, 5 years. 11

Reasons to Quit Card. 16

Number of Lifetime Puffs. 30

Tobacco Use Record. 32

Nicotine Blood Levels throughout the Day. 37

"Benefits of Smoking" and "Consequences of
Quitting". 50

Compare and Contrast Lists. 56

My Action Plan. 67

Nicotine Withdrawal and Coping Strategies Card. 91

Stress Graphic. 109

About the Author

As a former smoker, VJ Sleight knows how easy it is to stop smoking and how difficult it is to stay quit, even after receiving a cancer diagnosis. When she was 32, she was told she had breast cancer. While the doctors didn't suggest an association between her cancer and smoking, she would remain at high risk for a reoccurrence for the rest of her life as a smoker. This did motivate her to quit. If the cancer ever came back, she didn't want to guess that maybe, *"It was something I did to myself"*. She became a Queen of Quitting, by stopping smoking for at least three months, nine separate times.

Sleight gave her first Stop Smoking Workshop in 1990, one month after she put out her last cigarette. Since then, helping others become smoke-free has become a passion and personal mission. She has a Master's degree in Health Psychology and Behavioral Medicine, and has been trained at the Mayo Clinic as a Tobacco Treatment Specialist. She is a passionate speaker; traveling nationally to educate health care providers on how to effectively motivate patients to quit and smokers on how to develop a successful Plan. She offers both individual and group counseling in Southern California. As a cancer advocate, she is active locally as a Legislative Ambassador for the American Cancer Society Cancer Action Network. She is the Chairperson of the "Coalition for Tobacco-Free Communities Serving Riverside County" and a member of "Tobacco Use Reduction Now" in San Bernardino County.

In 2010, VJ didn't have to wonder if becoming smoke-free was the right decision when she received a second cancer diagnosis, instead she felt relief at having quit when she did. If she had continued smoking, the cancer may have come back sooner, been more aggressive and she might not be here today. The recurrence has only escalated her desire to help smokers who want to quit, get the resources they need.

Email: VJSleight@gmail.com

Website: www.VJSleight.com